Thriving with PCOS

Thriving with PCOS

Lifestyle Strategies to Successfully Manage Polycystic Ovary Syndrome

Kelly Morrow-Baez

ROWMAN & LITTLEFIELD
Lanham • Boulder • New York • London

Published by Rowman & Littlefield
A wholly owned subsidiary of The Rowman & Littlefield Publishing Group, Inc.
4501 Forbes Boulevard, Suite 200, Lanham, Maryland 20706
www.rowman.com

Unit A, Whitacre Mews, 26-34 Stannary Street, London SE11 4AB

British Library Cataloguing in Publication Information Available

Library of Congress Cataloging-in-Publication Data
Names: Morrow-Baez, Kelly, 1976– author.
Title: Thriving with PCOS : lifestyle strategies to successfully manage
   polycystic ovary syndrome / Kelly Morrow-Baez.
Description: Lanham : Rowman & Littlefield, [2018] | Includes bibliographical
   references and index.
Identifiers: LCCN 2017029198 (print) | LCCN 2017030654 (ebook) |
   ISBN 9781538108055 (electronic) | ISBN 9781538108048 (cloth : alk. paper)
Subjects: | MESH: Polycystic Ovary Syndrome—therapy | Polycystic Ovary
   Syndrome—psychology | Healthy Lifestyle | Health Behavior
Classification: LCC RG480.S7 (ebook) | LCC RG480.S7 (print) | NLM WP 320 |
   DDC 618.1/1—dc23
LC record available at https://lccn.loc.gov/2017029198

∞™ The paper used in this publication meets the minimum requirements of
American National Standard for Information Sciences—Permanence of Paper for
Printed Library Materials, ANSI/NISO Z39.48-1992.

Printed in the United States of America

To my mom,
who always told me I'd write a book.
And to my dad,
who gave me the determination to go out and do it.

Contents

Foreword

Sherry A. Ross

After twenty-five years practicing as an OBGYN, I can tell you that women who have some or all of the symptoms of polycystic ovary syndrome are completely confused. What is PCOS? How is it treated? What does it mean for them down the road? Unfortunately, women with this syndrome are also more prone to serious medical conditions than the average population. But in reading this book, you will learn how to avoid these common medical conditions with healthy-living strategies through diet, exercise, cognitive behavioral therapy, mindfulness, a regular sleep schedule, and being proactive in your medical care.

What is wonderful about this book is that Dr. Kelly Morrow-Baez has personally experienced the signs, symptoms, and frustrations associated with this chronic syndrome and here offers doable lifestyle remedies to help you navigate this syndrome. Her approach is proactive, holistic, and realistic. She reinforces three basic mantras—motivation, mind-set, and mindfulness—to guide you through managing PCOS. She answers the question *Why me?* when it comes to accepting your diagnosis of PCOS. You can handle and conquer the diagnosis if you follow her path of dealing with and accepting PCOS.

Many women with PCOS have a challenging time losing weight and tend to be overweight or obese. Not only is this frustrating, but it can also be isolating and depressing. Kelly helps you take control of your body, showing you how to eat foods that are plant-based, nutrient-rich, fresh, and unprocessed, along with healthy fats, and otherwise implement an ideal diet that becomes a lifelong diet strategy. She understands full well that controlling your weight also helps control other symptoms of PCOS—like irregular periods, excess hair growth, and acne.

If you are among the 5–10 percent of women who suffer from symptoms of PCOS, know that there are many treatment options available. As Kelly explains in great detail, healthy living and thinking holistically may be your best prescription. She assists you in developing healthy-lifestyle strategies and aids you in developing new habits, like personal journaling, that will bring you results.

Any woman suffering from PCOS could use a knowledgeable "wellness dream team" of experts, including a gynecologist and nutritionist, and Kelly gives you some invaluable suggestions for putting together your own care team, which, when combined with your own newly adopted healthy lifestyle choices, will take you far on the road to successfully managing your PCOS. The good news is that there are great treatments to control the symptoms caused by PCOS, and adapting certain lifestyle behaviors will help avoid some of the long-term medical diseases. While there is no cure for PCOS, effective treatment depends on the symptoms you are experiencing and your commitment to meeting medical interventions with a proactive lifestyle strategy. Treating each symptom separately will depend on how disruptive each one is in your life and daily routine.

Kelly's recommendations make sense, are doable, and free you from the confusion associated with a diagnosis of PCOS. Her journal questions following each chapter will help you focus on ways to improve your mind-set and develop a deeper understanding of your roadblocks to wellness.

Dr. Kelly Morrow-Baez is a PCOS survivor, a realist, and a woman who can walk you through life understanding and accepting a diagnosis of PCOS. Best of all, Kelly provides hope for managing all the obstacles too often overlooked by health-care providers. Healthy living and focusing on the positive is your best treatment in dealing with a PCOS diagnosis.

Learn and live through Kelly's supportive tools and strategies for healthy living and refining your own personal story so you can live life thriving with PCOS. As Kelly simply puts it, *the time is now to take control of your health*. Proactive self-care is possible and is the solution to not letting PCOS ruin your life. Being a consistent partner in your health is half the battle, and the strategies in this book will help you make that a reality.

Sherry A. Ross, MD
Obstetrician-gynecologist, women's health expert, and author of
She-ology: The Definitive Guide to Women's Intimate Health. Period.

1

❖ ❖

You Have PCOS; Now What?

THE BIG PICTURE

When you are first diagnosed with polycystic ovary syndrome (PCOS), it will be a relief to have confirmation that the symptoms you have been experiencing are real and meaningful. However, the diagnosis is just the starting point. If you are like many women, the first thing you will probably do is an Internet search, and that will lead you to a dismal list of symptoms and treatment options. You'll likely see diagrams of cystic ovaries and ads for laser hair removal. You might also read scary stories of infertility and diabetes, and you'll most definitely hear that it's next to impossible to lose weight.

Then there's the reality: that you are not alone. There is life after a PCOS diagnosis, and, to be honest, it's just plain normal.

WHY I WROTE THIS BOOK

The purpose of this book is not to replace the advice or intervention of your doctor. The purpose of this book is to help clarify the benefits of a healthy lifestyle as it relates to PCOS and demystify the process of making the necessary changes. When it comes to managing the syndrome, I believe that the combination of healthy lifestyle change and medical intervention is the most powerful changemaker.

While I can give you my personal experience regarding medical interventions, I am by no means stating that one thing is better than another. That is between you and your medical provider.

My professional background is in mental health, not medicine. I am writing this book because I've noticed a distinct gap between diagnosis and successful lifestyle change. Have you ever wondered why, when there are so many perfectly wonderful diet and exercise plans out there, people still struggle to lose weight? I believe there is a missing piece to the wellness puzzle—one that gets lost in the visual noise of the online fitness world. That missing piece is the psychology of change. I'll show you how to flip the switch and turn on your lasting motivation so that you reach your long-term health goals.

Success in any lifestyle plan comes down to three things:

1. *Motivation*—the desire to change or accomplish something
2. *Mind-set*—believing that growth and change are possible in any situation
3. *Mindfulness*—being aware of the present moment, no matter what you're doing

My goal is to break down these three concepts into tools that you can use to design your healthiest life. I can promise you that once you know the backstory to wellness, you will thrive as a woman with PCOS. If you want something different, you have to do something different. That difference is in this book.

My reasons for writing this book weren't all clinical. Some were personal. I was diagnosed with endometriosis at age nineteen and PCOS when I was twenty-three. The Internet was not as robust a resource then as it is now, but what I did find online scared me. I asked my doctor for metformin, which was the medical treatment of choice at the time. He flatly refused and said that I simply needed to go and lose weight. I felt shamed, because he said it as if I had never heard of the idea, as if it were a simple choice. I left his office feeling defeated and overwhelmed. I had read along the way that cutting out sugar and being more active were helpful, so that's where I began. I was in college, so I had access to a super gym, but I always felt out of place there. I usually went in the off hours so there wouldn't be so many people. I swam and did the elliptical. I lifted weights. I have a history of binge eating, but I started noticing the unhealthy food habits, although it was some time before I made any changes. This dipping-my-toe-into-the-water approach was exactly what I needed. The pounds started to come off, my clothes fit better, and my confidence soared. It didn't take a dramatic weight loss to get my symptoms under control, either. My Big Reason Why I was able to motivate myself was attached to my fear of the health consequences if I didn't get this under control, but there was another layer to my motivation: I wanted to look healthier. People define a healthy look in an infinite number of ways, but for me, I wanted to look like an athlete: slim, toned, and energetic. My starting point included none of those things, but as I started moving, I became increasingly focused on looking as fit and healthy as I felt.

A surprising benefit to achieving my health goals was that I became emotionally healthier too. My generalized anxiety disorder was kept in check, along with my insulin resistance. In this book you will learn how anxiety and insulin resistance are connected.

Healing myself from PCOS feels like a miracle and a blessing. When I discovered what worked, I felt that I was given my life back. Making weight loss more about good health and less about the number on the scale meant that my focus was on *living* and not on incessantly counting calories and carbs. I don't worry that PCOS is a lifelong syndrome, because the solution is a perfectly natural fit. I want to help you get your life back. I'm not talking about what you settle for, but rather the all-in-no-holds-barred life that is inherently yours.

While there is a seemingly infinite number of exercise and diet plans out there, none of them is of any use if you don't know how to put them into action in a way that will last. My answer to that gap between a doctor's diagnosis and total wellness is to help you develop an effective lifestyle strategy.

Diet and exercise advice that we see online and in magazines doesn't always cut it for women with PCOS. Crash diets and intense exercise plans aren't sustainable and can be counterproductive.

I'm in this for the long term because the syndrome is lifelong. Even living with PCOS that is in remission, it is an awareness that I have. When I got pregnant the first time, I didn't have very many symptoms of PCOS; I was fit and not overweight at all. Neither my doctor nor I gave much attention to my PCOS. I had a miscarriage. After the second miscarriage, my doctor decided to get more serious about treating my PCOS and put me on progesterone, which can help support the early stages of pregnancy.

My acne has always been present unless I was on a specific medication for it. During my pregnancies and while I was breastfeeding my children, I chose not to take any medication for fear it would hurt my baby somehow. I endured the pain and embarrassment of acne for nearly a decade before I talked to a doctor about my skin. Once prescribed, spironolactone was a miracle drug for me. Within three months of starting it, I had perfectly clear skin. That said, there is not a standard approach to treating PCOS-related cystic acne. What works for one woman might not work for the next.

Most of all, I want you to know this: There is hope with PCOS. You *can* get healthy. It likely won't come to you overnight, but it will definitely come. Release the image of yourself that has been altered by PCOS. You are at the beginning of a lifelong commitment to good health. Instead of emotional out-of-control eating, there will be empowered food choices. The *shoulds* in your internal dialogue will be replaced by an unwavering self-confidence. This is not to say that there won't be twists and turns along the way, but in this book I will show you how to navigate them so that you stay on track, becoming the healthiest version of yourself. I can't guarantee that you will be a size 2 fitness model, but I can promise that you will have a deeper understanding of PCOS and the mind-set to make better health a reality.

WHAT YOU NEED TO KNOW TO GET STARTED

The exact cause of PCOS is hotly debated among researchers. PCOS is a syndrome—or, rather, a collection of symptoms triggered by the way the body responds to insulin and androgens. *PCOS* is actually a misnomer. In fact, serious talks are underway in the medical community to more accurately label the condition as metabolic reproductive syndrome. True, the vast majority of women with this condition have cysts on their ovaries, but some do not. The current approach to diagnosis is the Rotterdam criteria. To say that you have PCOS, you have to have at least two out of three features: no ovulation or infrequent ovulation, elevated testosterone levels that can result in hirsutism, and/or male-pattern hair loss, along with multiple cysts on the ovaries as confirmed by an ultrasound.[1] Because symptoms vary so much among women with PCOS, researchers are debating the possibility of breaking PCOS into different types rather than tallying up a list of symptoms.

There is a hereditary aspect to PCOS, so it is entirely possible that your mother or grandmother had it, even if they were never diagnosed. According to a study in Australia, up to 70 percent of women with PCOS are never diagnosed.[2]

PCOS usually starts in the teen years, around the time of the first menstrual cycle. Symptoms can become more distressing over time and can significantly worsen when a woman gains weight. This is troublesome, because weight gain is a slippery slope. An increase in weight causes symptoms to worsen and creates more insulin resistance, making it harder to lose weight. If this sounds familiar, then it's time to step off that particular ride. This book is designed to give you the backstory to PCOS and guide you on the path toward managing this syndrome. Ultimately, you will have all the information you need to achieve a lasting and lifelong transformation.

I believe that the best result comes from joining medical interventions with new, healthy living habits. By doing all the good we can do with lifestyle changes, the medications are more effective and at possibly lower doses. And lower doses means fewer side effects. If you are choosing to heal your PCOS without medical interventions, this book will still be helpful, and I have no judgments about that approach. Keep in mind that you are absolutely in control. You decide which lifestyle strategies you implement, and you are in control of your long-term commitment to them. It is not an all-or-nothing experience. When it comes to making healthy changes, one of the most dangerous mind-set mistakes is that we "should" on ourselves. Even if the thing you *should* do is positive—like exercising every day—it is an unhelpful criticism best left out of your mind-set practice. Criticism is poison for any motivation. Your best bet is to become aware of the shoulds in your life, whether from your doctor, your spouse, or yourself. Dig deep, and ask, *Why am I resisting making healthy changes?*

Whatever you decide, whether it's medical intervention or not, understand that your plan and even your goals will evolve over time. PCOS is a lifelong syndrome, but we are not a set-it-and-forget-it species. Make a commitment to evaluate and reevaluate whenever you lose sight of your goals.

INSULIN RESISTANCE 101

Up to 70 percent of women with PCOS are also insulin resistant.[3] Insulin is a naturally occurring hormone secreted by the pancreas that acts as a doorman for sugar to enter the cells. When a person is insulin resistant, the doorman is essentially working with a jammed door, and sugar can't get into the cells to be used as energy. Because the cells aren't getting enough sugar, they assume no one is there to hold the door open, so they send signals to the pancreas to send more insulin to open that door. More insulin doesn't improve effectiveness; it just wears out the pancreas, which is why PCOS often results in type 2 diabetes.

There are many secondary effects from insulin resistance—a collection of symptoms that go beyond the Rotterdam criteria and make up the syndrome that we know as PCOS.

Common symptoms of insulin resistance include:

absence or irregularity of periods
heavy, painful periods
acne and/or oily skin
loss of scalp hair
obesity or overweight
elevated testosterone
excess hair on face or body

WHY ALL THE FUSS ABOUT OVARIES?

Ovaries are designed to take turns releasing an egg each month. If the egg doesn't get fertilized, it gets shed in a menstrual cycle. For women with PCOS, lack of regular periods is typical. Cysts can form when the egg starts to be released, like it would for a normal menstrual cycle, but then gets clogged in the follicle. Cysts are like a pimple in your ovary. It is not uncommon for both ovaries to have numerous cysts due to the eggs not being released; however, not all women who have PCOS will have cystic ovaries. Discomfort levels as a result of cystic ovaries vary from nonexistent to excruciating. If you experience sudden severe pain in the lower left or right part of your body, call your doctor right away.

Because ovaries produce estrogen and testosterone, they have an effect that goes beyond the reproductive system and can wreak havoc on the whole body when they aren't functioning properly. You can think of a woman's monthly cycle like a web: if one part of it is disturbed or damaged, then it can have far-reaching effects on the whole system.

TESTOSTERONE

Many women get nervous when they learn their testosterone levels are elevated. Keep in mind that, while testosterone plays a larger role in men's bodies, it is a normal part of a woman's cocktail of hormones. Normal levels of testosterone in a woman's body support energy, mood, reproductive health, and libido. Elevated levels of testosterone resulting from insulin resistance can cause excess facial hair and acne around the jawline (basically where a man's beard would be; more on acne in chapter 10). It can also cause weight gain, balding, or thinning of hair.

FREE VERSUS TOTAL TESTOSTERONE

The two ways to measure testosterone are assessing the total testosterone or just the free testosterone. Free testosterone is the measurement of testosterone that is "unbound" and active in your body. Unfortunately, just a small amount of additional testosterone is enough to disrupt the menstrual cycle.

There are several ways in which we can attempt to reduce free testosterone. They have not all been thoroughly researched and proven to work; however, they might be worth considering. Always check with your doctor before making any changes to medication or supplements.

Birth control pills—There are numerous options for birth control pills, which contain female hormones that can offset the effect of testosterone. Talk to your doctor about any side effects.

Metformin—This medication reduces blood sugar in the body, which reduces insulin, thus lowering testosterone.

Spironolactone—This and other antiandrogen medications have been found to reduce testosterone. Spironolactone was originally developed as a diuretic for people with heart disease. While it is not terribly effective in that regard, it is quite effective in the treatment of excess facial hair and cystic acne.

Adjusting diet—Limiting simple carbs that spike your blood sugar can be helpful. Replacing them with complex carbohydrates like oatmeal, sweet potatoes, and beans will give you the energy you need in a way that is more "time released."

Switching to soy—Introducing products like tofu and tempeh to your diet can be helpful, as these foods contain phytoestrogens, a plant form of estrogen. It has been suggested that phytoestrogens potentially offset the effect of testosterone.

Myoinositol—This new supplement for the treatment of PCOS has been found to be effective in treating insulin resistance, anxiety, and testosterone levels.

WEIGHT LOSS AND PCOS

Up to 80 percent of women with PCOS are overweight.[4] One reason women with PCOS have such a hard time with weight loss is because their insulin levels are generally higher than the general female population. In addition to getting glucose into the cells, insulin has a secondary job of storing glucose in the form of fat. If your insulin is higher, yet resistant to doing its job of getting glucose to the cells for immediate energy, then it has plenty of glucose to store as fat.[5]

You may have heard from your doctor that your BMI is too high. BMI stands for *body mass index*. It's calculated by dividing your weight in kilograms by your height in centimeters squared. In case you're curious, BMI calculators are all over the Internet. BMI is often used because it's quick and simple and looks good in a medical chart. However, it does not differentiate between fat and muscle. (At his fittest, Arnold Schwarzenegger had a BMI in the obese category!) Better health stats to watch are blood pressure, cholesterol, resting heart rate, and body fat percentage. Also helpful is simply monitoring how you *feel* and even how your clothes fit.

Insulin also stimulates appetite. Women with PCOS often have intense cravings, and many experience binge-eating behavior. A study was done that compared the response to images of junk food after a sugar drink. Women who do not have PCOS had no reaction to the images of food. It didn't excite them in any way or trigger cravings. Essentially, their body was clear that they had consumed enough sugar and did not want anything more. On the other hand, women who have PCOS were given the sugar drink and then shown images of junk food, and researchers found that sections of the brain were stimulated as evidenced by a magnetic resonance imaging (MRI). This is why it is so important for women with PCOS to avoid sugar. Eating sugar causes more intense sugar cravings.

Another reason it is easy to gain weight as a woman with PCOS is that our metabolism is significantly slower! Your *basal metabolic rate* is the number of calories your body needs to carry out basic functions. For women without PCOS, the average basal metabolic rate is about 1,800 calories. For women with PCOS, that number is about 1,450 calories. If a woman has insulin resistance along with PCOS—which is usually the case—then that number is even lower.[6] Women with PCOS tend to store fat in their midsection, which is the most dangerous area, especially as women age, due to the increased risk of heart disease associated with this fat.[7]

HOW TO STIMULATE INSULIN SENSITIVITY

While most people make the mistake of focusing on which exercise to do or which supplement to take in order to lose weight or gain fertility, the foundation of PCOS is insulin resistance. In order to have a therapeutic effect from any of your efforts, it's important to focus on that central issue. Medications like metformin can be useful; however, this is a conversation to have with your doctor, as there are undesirable side effects as well. Lifestyle management combined with medical interventions produces the best effect.

In this book we explore and expand on these strategies to reverse insulin resistance:

Cardio—Thirty minutes of cardio every day with just enough intensity to slightly elevate your heart rate will burn off the stress hormone cortisol and excess glucose and improve mood.

Weight training—More muscle means more places for the insulin to store and use glucose. One of the benefits of having PCOS is that we tend to put on muscle a bit more easily than other women (but don't worry— you'd still have to try awfully hard to get that bodybuilder look).

Stress management—Stress creates cortisol, and cortisol blocks the effectiveness of insulin.

Weight loss—Easier said than done, but the body perceives excess adipose tissue (fat) much in the same way it would were you consistently eating high-fat meals.

Avoiding bad fats—Limit saturated fats, which are found mostly in meats and in some nuts and seeds, and eliminate trans fats altogether. (More on this in chapter 2.)

Getting adequate sleep.

Remember, this is not a one-off experience. Being healthy when you have PCOS requires that you develop these strategies into a lasting lifestyle. Don't fight your PCOS. Instead, lead the ongoing dance with insulin resistance.

THINKING HOLISTICALLY

Many women make the mistake of trying to extinguish the symptoms of PCOS without getting to the core of the issue. Fighting the symptoms and not the source results in the medical equivalent of wellness Whac-A-Mole. This can lead to additional stress and feelings of hopelessness. It's a challenge to accept the idea that such a distinct medical diagnosis with very real medical symptoms would have something as vague as "lifestyle change" as the solution. The answer isn't to search for a cure, because the reality is that there is no cure for PCOS. The goal of lifestyle change is to keep PCOS in *remission*. As you read, you may have a hard time believing that this sort of solution, lifestyle change, could really work, but it most definitely can. Often a doctor will be willing to prescribe something like metformin or birth control pills. All medicines have their pros and cons, and it's up to each individual to choose to medicate (or not) with the guidance of their doctor. I want to be clear: Doctors aren't the enemy—they want to help you in any way they can. Unfortunately, the training doctors receive on lifestyle strategies for better health are secondary to their clinical work, and current trends in managed care limit the amount of time they can spend with you to explain it all. The bottom line is that there is no cure for PCOS, so if you want to make huge, lasting, and healthy changes, you have to put in the effort to design a lifestyle that supports your goals by working *alongside* any medical intervention you choose. Otherwise a pill is nothing more than a Band-Aid.

Sometimes people get frustrated when I talk about lifestyle change as a way to manage PCOS, but PCOS is a syndrome, not an infection, so the only solution is to take *consistent* steps in the direction of your health. That is easier said than done, but by knowing the psychology behind it, your motivation and focus will be empowered and energized. You may worry that you're not up to the task, your life isn't settled enough, and you're compelled to accept what is and give up. I hear you, but I want to offer you an alternative.

The concepts I've outlined are from a combination of personal and professional experience topped off with hundreds of hours of research. There is no quick fix. This is a sustainable holistic approach that is completely possible to achieve.

I do not want to override the advice or direction of your doctor. The purpose of this book is to pick up where the diagnosis leaves off and help you partner better with your doctor. I believe that when you do your part to match the medical interventions with lifestyle changes you get the best result. Unfortunately, I see far too many women who are mystified, confused, and unfortunately uninformed about the importance and benefit of lifestyle changes for PCOS. They rely only on medical interventions to solve this complex issue. While medical interventions are wonderful, they often have side effects. Also, if the medicine has to work against the issues inherent in PCOS coupled with poor diet and sedentary lifestyle, then the medicine is going to have to work harder. That leaves you with a trade-off: higher dose or reduced effectiveness? If you are consistently eating a healthy diet, one that doesn't spike your blood sugar, metformin will reduce the sugars that are in your body, and you will get a better overall result. If you manage your stress and your sleep and anything else that would trigger insulin resistance, then the medication doesn't have to work as hard as it would if you were eating junk food and living in a state of constant stress.

In these pages you will learn and understand the lifestyle strategies, the mind-set, the motivation, and all of the psychological pieces comprising a healthy lifestyle that will help you, in partnership with your medical doctor, get the most positive and healthy result. The reason many women don't make healthy lifestyle changes is because they have no idea what that means. Doctors don't have time to explain, and so women can come away from their appointments confused, anxious, overwhelmed, and desperate for help. There are some incredible and scary effects of mismanaged PCOS.

I don't have a product to sell you. What I want to share with you is a strategy for a healthy mind-set that you can apply to your own life. This is not a one-size-fits-all solution. I want you to apply this to your own life: your own preferences, your own schedule, your own culture. In this way, it becomes a lifestyle that is as sustainable as it is healthy. So try to keep a pen and paper handy as you go through the book. This is especially important with the diet and exercise sections. When you're crafting a lifestyle strategy, it's important to know that it will not be a fixed plan. It must be flexible and adjustable. There will be times in your life when this is easier and other times when it's harder. Starting out on a healthy-lifestyle plan is a lot like starting a new job: a lot of mental energy is spent just getting through activities that soon will become automatic.

Imagine yourself being the star patient. Imagine walking into the doctor's office for a checkup, and suddenly your weight is significantly lower than it was on your last visit, and your blood sugar levels are within normal limits, your cycles are regular, and your acne has cleared. Not only that, but your anxiety has also been replaced with confidence, and your chronic exhaustion has been replaced with boundless energy. All the indicators of PCOS are managed. That reality is much closer than you think. Working through the suggestions in this book will show you how to achieve total health.

As I mentioned, I am not a medical doctor. I am most concerned with your mind-set, motivation, and understanding of what it's going to take to get you healthy. I want to help you do everything that is within your power so that you are healthy in body, mind, and spirit. The reason it's important to create a plan that is enduring is because PCOS is a syndrome, meaning that it is not going away. There is no cure. So we have to meet that reality with a long-term solution.

WHAT CAUSES PCOS?

The reality is that there is no known cause of PCOS. Research indicates that there is a genetic predisposition for the syndrome. If your mother or sister has it, then there is a good chance you will have it. Another reality is that there seems to be a threshold for development of the syndrome that is crossed when a woman gains a significant amount of weight or develops inflammation due to chronic stress. While the genetic link is well documented, this trigger, extra weight, could be linked to cultural trends within families that combine with a genetic predisposition to result in PCOS.[8] Weight gain can trigger PCOS in women who have a predisposition for the syndrome. While a single cause has yet to be identified, there are theories about how this happens.

PCOS AND MENOPAUSE

Because PCOS involves the release of eggs from ovaries, many women wonder whether their symptoms will go away when they reach menopause.

In one sense, it's an understandable question, especially when the focus often seems to be on ovaries and fertility. When you reach menopause you stop releasing eggs, and the hormones responsible for reproduction change. Unfortunately, you don't get a free pass once you reach meno-pause. Testosterone does decrease, and it seems to reach normal levels by about age sixty-one; however, women with PCOS still have an increased risk of the inflammatory and cardiovascular problems that normally become more prevalent with age.

THE GOOD NEWS

Women who have PCOS reach menopause later in life compared to women who do not have the syndrome. Women with PCOS also experience more regular periods as they age due to the decrease of testosterone over time and are more likely to be able to conceive later in life. Hot flashes and night sweats also tended to be less severe in women who have PCOS.

THE BAD NEWS

Not much else changes. The rates of excess hair growth are still higher than in women who don't have PCOS at a rate of 64 percent to 9 percent.[9]

Heart disease is the number one killer of women, and if you have PCOS, your chances of developing heart disease are elevated. This is a significant concern as you age. Women with PCOS have been found to have higher levels of C-reactive protein (CRP), which is a measurement of inflammation. In addition, women with PCOS are found to have higher triglycerides and lower HDL (the good cholesterol). Insulin resistance and other metabolic markers are also likely to persist.

The news isn't all bad. In fact, studies have shown that PCOS-related health issues are really more a reality for women who are obese but not so much in overweight or lean women who have PCOS.

CALL TO ACTION

Get healthy. Now. Doing as much as you can for yourself now is an investment in your health that will pay dividends later on. The book you're holding is designed to give you a roadmap for a healthy strategy you can use throughout your life.

> The moment you take responsibility for everything in your life is the moment you can change anything in your life.
>
> —Hal Elrod

I've walked this path, and I'm excited to walk it with you too. You can do this. Let's get started.

JOURNALING TIPS

At the end of each chapter, there will be some journaling questions that will help you get clear on how to make ideas become reality in your life. You might feel inclined to skip over the journaling parts and "just think about them." Here's why you shouldn't do that:

- Writing slows down your thoughts and gives them structure, which creates mindfulness.
- The act of writing signals to your brain, *This is important*, which will then trigger the reticular activating system (RAS) of your brain to look for opportunities throughout the day to help you achieve that goal.
- Some of us use food as a coping strategy for stress, anxiety, and resentment. You must replace one coping strategy with another— otherwise, you're just running on willpower, which is fickle at best. Journaling is an effective way to replace one coping strategy with another, healthier one.

JOURNAL QUESTIONS

One of the most powerful ways to maintain and nurture motivation through the ups and downs of life is to get crystal clear about your *why*. The answer has to be deep—at the core level. For help finding your why, go to your journal and play what I call the click-down exercise:

1. Why do you want to manage your PCOS with lifestyle changes?
   o Take your answer to question 1, and ask yourself why you want that.

o Take *that* answer, and ask yourself why you want that.

o Keep going until you get to the core. Your core. The answer that makes you furious or gives you goose bumps or even makes you cry. That's your why. Write it down, and keep it where you can see it as you create your healthy lifestyle.

2. How do you feel about managing PCOS with lifestyle changes?
3. What lifestyle changes do you want to make to manage your PCOS?
4. How would you describe what getting healthy means to you?

2

❖ ❖

Diet

Eating to Heal

The goal of a PCOS diet is to reduce insulin resistance. The way to do that is to fuel the body with food that will keep your body nourished, your metabolism stoked, and your mind satisfied.

SUGAR CONSUMPTION AND PCOS

Many people confuse carbohydrates and sugar. Sugar is a type of carbohydrate. We need quality carbohydrates, but as women with PCOS we don't tolerate sugar as well. Limit sugar and prepackaged carbohydrates. I didn't say *eliminate* sugar. No food is off-limits forever (unless you have an allergic reaction to it). The reason for this is because if you swear off a food, you're going to put an enormous amount of energy into resisting it, which actually puts more mental focus on that food you're trying to avoid. The trick is to understand how and why your body reacts to sugar and adjust your diet accordingly.

If you are going to eat sugar, that's okay, as long as it is in moderation. You've probably heard that before, but what does it mean? At the core of moderation you want to choose the sugar that satisfies your cravings but in limited amounts so that you don't set off the need for more. There are some common high-sugar foods that would be better left out so that you can make room for an indulgence that is more satisfying. Also, many women will report that they have "trigger foods" that will set off overeating. Take a moment now to consider your trigger foods and high-sugar foods you might not miss terribly. What could you replace those foods with so that you get the most pleasure out of your indulgence?

A word about sugar-free sweets: Very often the sugar-replacement ingredient is maltitol or some other sugar alcohol. These ingredients can wreak havoc on your digestive system and result in severe bloating, excessive gas, and diarrhea. Instead, opt for fruit or natural sugar-free sweeteners like stevia to sweeten your favorite treats.

I spend a lot of time on sugar because it's important to get it right. Any sugar you eat will float around in your bloodstream, waiting to be used or put away. Sugar is inflammatory, which can lead to all sorts of problems:

Inflammation can lead to cardiovascular disease.
It can contribute to infertility.
It can make acne worse.

As discussed in chapter 1, insulin resistance prevents sugar from getting into your cells. When cells don't get enough sugar, they assume there isn't enough insulin out there to get the job done, so they send signals to the pancreas to send more insulin. The reason lifestyle change is so important is because eventually the pancreas will become exhausted from overuse and give out, resulting in type 2 diabetes.

Don't be surprised if you fall off the wagon from time to time. That's not failure. Failure is an experience, not an identity. So if you go overboard with the doughnuts in the break room, that's okay. Stay aware of how it made you feel. Did you get tired? Start to feel anxious? Did you get a headache?

Many women have spent so much time feeling crummy that it's hard to notice these effects because they are used to feeling bad. Take the time to notice them. Are you feeling sluggish? Anxious? Is your thinking not as sharp as you think it should be? Are you walking around in a mental fog?

BETTER CARBOHYDRATE CHOICES

You may be wondering what carbs you *can* eat. A helpful way to get ideas is to look at the glycemic index, or GI, the standard of measurement indicating how much a particular food raises your blood sugar. There are carbs (like pretzels, cookies, and frosting) that hit your bloodstream in a rush, leaving you feeling terrible; these foods are high on the GI. Then there are others that enter your bloodstream more gradually, with a slower burn; these are lower-GI foods. The lower the GI, the less your blood sugar is elevated by them, and the better you will feel after eating them.

While in general I'm a big proponent of diet tracking, these apps have one major flaw: they see a carb as a carb. There is no distinction between 50 carbs of cake or 50 carbs of sweet potatoes; yet the effect these have on your body and the way you feel can vary dramatically. The choice is up to you, and, while you might not want to swear off cake, you do want to develop an awareness of what foods will help you feel stronger, more clear-headed, and more energetic. Filling your allotment of carbs with lower-GI carbs will do just that.

Perspective is everything, and that is true for making healthier diet choices as well. Instead of focusing on a list of foods to avoid, look at everything that you *can* eat. Explore recipes with those ingredients. Think about how you will feel when you feel good.

The average food craving lasts about fifteen minutes. If you can delay your response to a food for fifteen minutes, chances are that the craving will pass. Even if it doesn't, you have a lot more awareness and control over the situation and will be much more likely to make a healthier choice, or at least indulge in moderation.

FINDING A SUSTAINABLE EATING PATTERN

Many actors will say that the harder roles to play are the ones where the character is basically normal, whereas the wild, bizarre, very out-there characters are actually easier to conjure. The same is true when it comes to making healthy food choices a part of your daily lifestyle. Most people get excited about fad diets because they are so different that it's easier to lock onto a major aspect of that particular fad. The lifestyle change you actually need to get *healthy* isn't weird, extreme, or crazy. You don't have to live off broth or forage like a caveman; you don't have to eat baby food. You just have to be aware of how your body responds to food and eat accordingly. The bottom line is that diets don't have to be extreme. In fact, they *shouldn't* be extreme. The reason so many people struggle with healthy eating is because it is so normal that it borders on boring.

The beautiful thing about the human body is that, except in some rare circumstances, it is incredibly flexible and forgiving. To achieve better health, it's not necessary to follow any program to the letter. In fact, it's this resilience that allows eating habits to go from rigid, unattainable rules to a very achievable lifestyle change.

> **TIP:** When considering a diet, if it has a marketable, recognizable, or otherwise catchy name, and makes for good watercooler conversation, it's probably a fad, it may not be healthy, and it definitely won't be sustainable.
>
> Instead, go with a *normal* diet. Follow the general guidelines: stay away from processed foods (especially fast food), avoid unnecessary sugar such as in soda and prepackaged sweets, eat more vegetables, and limit processed carbs like white rice and white bread.

It's hard to believe that so moderate a change can have such powerful results. The power isn't in the diet as much as it is in the *consistency* of that diet. The consistency comes from mind-set.

Does that mean that a healthy, normal diet has to be boring? Absolutely not! Remember, the English language was created by various combinations of twenty-six letters. When you prepare food, the same idea holds true. The combinations are essentially limitless, so it never has to be boring.

Almost every woman with PCOS falls into one of two eating styles:

1. The first is the people who think they are eating well but are still gaining weight. For women with PCOS, this is entirely likely because the body can't process sugar like most people, so it's hard to compare your diet with everyone else's. Overeating sugar and processed carbohydrates can leave women with PCOS feeling cloudy-headed, sluggish, and malnourished.

   For this type of eater, the easiest solution is to download a food-tracking app and master it. Mind-set changes come before lifestyle changes. That is why so few people make healthy, lasting changes—they don't have the right mind-set going in! PCOS is a medical condition. Just like people with diabetes are healthier when they use the right tools to monitor their health, women with PCOS find that a diet tracker is a valuable tool to help determine what foods help create balance, nourishment, and wellness.

2. There is another group of women, and so often they are women with PCOS who know they are eating poorly but think lifestyle change is beyond their reach. Women with PCOS are particularly susceptible to this error in mind-set, and it's easy to understand why. In the list of PCOS symptoms, weight gain comes in at the top. Learning that weight gain and difficulty losing weight is part of the syndrome makes efforts to get healthy seem insurmountable. The bottom line is that it's not true; having PCOS doesn't sentence you to obesity. If there is a sense of powerlessness surrounding food, it is often accompanied with feeling rushed, stressed, and overwhelmed. This is where mind-set can transform your experience.

Women with PCOS need not be defined by their syndrome. The goal of this book is to give you the information and tools to create a lifestyle that allows you to thrive with PCOS.

Many people eat what they want and stay healthy. As a result, many women with PCOS feel cheated that they have to adjust their diet. They're thinking, *It's not fair*. And, quite frankly, they'd be right. Here's the question: Is it better to be right or to be healthy? When you release the need to be right, you free up tremendous energy to put toward sustaining healthy changes until they become a consistent habit.

BINGE EATING

Women with PCOS are at greater risk of binge eating disorder than the general population. In a study published by *The Lancet*, about one-third of women with PCOS also have binge eating disorder; however, the rate is likely higher than that because of underreporting.[1] Most women know that it is not a healthy behavior pattern, nor is it good for their bodies, and so they are unlikely to admit to it.

Binge eating typically has a purely psychological cause, but women with PCOS have a physical reason for it as well. Eating just a small amount of sugar triggers excess insulin to be released into the bloodstream, which causes intense cravings for sweets.

Many women will ask me whether they have binge eating disorder. This is a difficult question to answer, but the more helpful question to ask yourself is whether you are showing signs of binge eating behavior such as eating a large amount of food in a short amount of time and feeling guilty or ashamed afterward.

This is different from the regret you feel after overindulging at a holiday meal. If you're overeating with an emotional or upset feeling behind it and turning overeating into a coping strategy, then that is something to give more attention to. Other signs of binge eating include eating more than what is considered normal and doing so at least once a week for three months.

There is a typical cycle to binge eating, especially when it has a psychological antecedent. The stage for binge eating is set when there is a history of control, fighting, powerlessness, or shame that was formed around eating when you were a child. This can pull eating from a nutritional or cultural definition and put it into a more emotionally charged part of the psyche. At that point, binge eating turns into a go-to coping strategy.

During a binge, there is a pressure to eat with the intent to calm negative emotions. After a binge, you're likely to feel physically uncomfortable and emotionally remorseful. As a woman with insulin resistance, you are likely to feel sluggish, weak, and dizzy, with cloudy thinking. Shame and remorse perpetuate the cycle, because negative self-talk erodes self-esteem and the belief that you can make changes.

So if you have PCOS and you notice a pattern of binge eating behavior, it's helpful to keep in mind that binge eating is a cycle. Effective interventions are going to be focused on breaking that cycle, not just suppressing the act of overeating. It is virtually impossible to stop the cycle of binge eating with willpower alone.

Fortunately, certain behaviors can help end binge eating.

Exercise—Daily exercise can reduce depression and increase confidence and build self-esteem. It is a healthy coping strategy.
Setting boundaries—Learn to say no to what doesn't serve you.
Journaling—Write about your feelings.
Delaying for fifteen minutes—This creates a gap so that you can create an awareness of the source of the craving.

Binge eating can be hard to treat because it is obviously impossible to abstain from food. Instead, you will have to create more mindfulness about how you have been using food and how you want to use food going forward. *Are you feeding your PCOS or fighting it?* Redefining this new relationship with food can be exciting and open up your life in ways that you could never imagine.

YOUR EATING CULTURE

Whether you recognize it or not, there is a culture and a tradition surrounding our eating habits.

I am from the South. That gives me a culture from which my perspective is formed, but I am also aware of the family traditions and beliefs that I grew up with.

Some cultural beliefs are easier to alter than others. Remember that changing a behavior is not about insulting, judging, or turning your back on your family beliefs or culture. It's about making small, thoughtful changes in your life with the goal of improving your health and well-being. Once again, keep your choices simple, focused, and mindful. Choose one area at a time that feels okay to change.

I knew a Mexican woman who was struggling with depression and anxiety and desperately wanted to lose weight. She also had a cultural norm of enjoying a rich hot chocolate and a generous portion of bread just before bed. She was able to see this as a cultural norm but not a rule. She was able to make the shift from hot chocolate to hot tea, saving herself 200 calories but still maintaining the important part of that activity—a coming together of the family after a long day.

Describe your culture. What cultural or family traditions surrounding eating habits do you hold? Are there any parts of those habits that you might change in order to improve your health?

> **TIP:** I wouldn't focus on occasional events like Christmas dinner; focus instead on the daily habits and cultural norms that might be affecting your diet.

WHAT TO EAT

Why Can't I Just Have a List of Foods to Eat?

The problem with any diet plan that you are likely to see on the Internet is that it's not *yours*. My goal in this chapter is to lay out all of the information about diet and PCOS so that you can create a plan that fits in your life, schedule, culture, and preferences. The choice of what to eat is a very personal decision. Trying to follow another person's diet plan to the letter because that's how they got healthy is like pretending to be someone you're not. Chances are good that it's not going to be a good fit.

Macronutrients

You may have seen macros calculated in your diet tracker, broken into three categories: *protein*, *carbohydrates*, and *fat*. Developing an awareness of ideal macronutrient ratios can help you avoid cravings and get the nutrition you need. From a practical standpoint, you can use the idea of macros to help you decide to eat.

Protein is the one part of your diet that you absolutely must eat because it cannot be created within the body. Protein is built with components called *amino acids*, and they can be combined to make protein much in the way that we use letters to create words. There are twenty amino acids that can be combined to create everything the body needs to live, heal, and grow. As you eat protein, the amino acids are broken down into their individual building blocks so that they can be reassembled in any way necessary. This is one of the reasons why fasting is controversial. You need protein every day, but with a consistent protein deficit your body will start to pull amino acids from muscle in your body to try to meet the demand. This is what causes muscle wasting. Keep in mind that your heart is a muscle, and it's imperative that it stay as strong as possible for optimal health.

Nine of the twenty amino acids that you need are essential, meaning that they cannot be created in the body and must come from your diet. Proteins from animal sources contain all of the essential amino acids and are termed *complete proteins*. Proteins from plant sources are incomplete, so it is important to get protein from a variety of sources if you are on a plant-based diet.

As for carbohydrates, for women with PCOS, the goal is low sugar. Sugar is the first place to start when you're changing your eating habits, because eating sugar triggers your brain into wanting more. Despite what you may have heard, carbohydrates are not the enemy. The key is to understand which carbohydrates provide a useful source of energy and which will spike your blood sugar. So before you swear off all carbohydrates, let's take a look at the main types.

Complex carbohydrates are ideal for a healthy body and lend themselves to a more stable blood-sugar level. Because of their complexity, it takes longer for the body to break those types of carbohydrates down into glucose, so it results in a slower release of glucose into the bloodstream over time. Examples of complex carbohydrates include sweet potatoes, beans, green vegetables, rolled oats, and whole-grain bread.

Simple carbohydrates have a basic design and can quickly be converted into glucose. Cakes, icing, pasta, and candy are all examples of simple carbohydrates. When there is too much sugar in the bloodstream on a regular basis, it can cause inflammation, insulin resistance, weight gain, and high blood pressure and can lead to kidney disease. In addition to the physical effects, eating simple carbohydrates has been found to trigger binge eating behavior in women with PCOS.

As for the final macronutrient, fat, the type of fat you eat matters. Knowing the differences can help you make healthier choices.[2]

Saturated fat is commonly found in meat, and this fat can raise cholesterol and increase your risk for heart disease. Low-carb diets tend to result in an increase in saturated fat consumption because most people meet the high demand for protein by increasing the amount of meat they eat. This puts women with PCOS at an even greater risk of heart disease.

Trans fat should not be eaten at all. There is such a strong link between heart disease, obesity, and trans fats that US legislation has been passed to require that trans fat be placed on the nutritional information in food packaging. The legislation goes even further to require food companies to eliminate trans fat from all food products in 2018. We typically see trans fats in fried foods and prepackaged baked goods.

Unsaturated fat is the healthiest of the fats; however, due to its dense calorie load, even this type of fat should be eaten in moderation. Switching from saturated fats to unsaturated fats has been shown to lower LDL cholesterol levels and reduce the risk of heart disease. Unsaturated fats can be separated into *polyunsaturated fats* and *monounsaturated fats*. Polyunsaturated fats are liquid at room temperature and in the refrigerator. This includes sesame oil, safflower oil, and corn oil. Sources of monounsaturated fats include olive oil and peanut oils, which are liquid at room temperature but tend to thicken in cooler temperatures.

It's important for women to manage their fat intake because the calorie count can add up quickly. Saturated fat can contribute to higher cholesterol levels and to heart disease. Excess fat, sugar, and processed-carbohydrate intake can also lead to nonalcoholic fatty liver disease (NAFLD). Women with PCOS are more likely to develop NAFLD, but when it is addressed quickly with diet and lifestyle change it is reversible.

Hidden Sugars

Avoiding sugar is easier said than done. One of my biggest frustrations with prepackaged foods and restaurant foods is the amount of hidden sugar; however, other foods you don't think of as "sweet" can also have a high amount of sugar. If you're eating something sweet, then you know that it has sugar, and you can make your decision from there. Unfortunately, salty and savory foods can be packed with sugar as well.

And you might not think about dairy being sugar-laden, but, actually, the cow's milk we drink so much of was not designed for human consumption; it was designed to grow a baby cow very quickly. There is a surprising amount of simple sugar, called *lactose*, in most milk products. Because it is a simple sugar, lactose is broken down into glucose very easily and can spike your blood sugar. Many people have also found that dairy makes their acne worse. A variety of plant-based alternatives to dairy can be found in almost every supermarket. Cashew milk, soy milk, and coconut milk are all good alternatives that can be used in cooking as well. Just make sure to get the unsweetened varieties.

Besides in prepackaged foods and dairy products, also watch out for added sugar in the following:

> *Condiments*—Barbeque sauce, stir-fry sauces, and ketchup all have hidden sugars that can add up quickly.
> *Bread*—It's not just the cinnamon-raisin bread we have to worry about! Not only are most breads high in carbohydrates, but they can also have hidden sugars in them that will make the impact to your blood sugar levels worse.
> *Alcohol*—Like bread, alcohol is frequently high in carbohydrates. Dry wines like cabernet sauvignon and pinot grigio have a reduced impact, but many women with PCOS report feeling intoxicated faster than their peers who do not have PCOS.

Learning to Like Vegetables

You know that vegetables are a big part of getting healthy. They have loads of nutrients, and as long as they are prepared without too much cheese, oil, or meat, you can really fill up on them without worrying about going over your calorie allotment.

But what do you do if the only vegetable you can tolerate is a potato? Give these suggestions a try:

You don't have to eat vegetables (yet). Start the first week or so simply replacing your processed-food snacks with fresh fruit.

Stop saying you don't like vegetables. Maybe you haven't found the one you like yet. This small shift in mind set is powerful.

Start small. Snag a bite of a vegetable off your friend's plate.

Each week, choose a vegetable you can tolerate. Experiment with it about once a day.

Try veggies in soup.

Hide them in smoothies.

Explore recipes. While raw carrot or cucumber sticks are wonderful (really), many cooking websites let you search for recipes by ingredient. I like Allrecipes because it allows you to include or exclude certain ingredients and narrow results by time to prepare, meal, and dish type.[3]

Consider whether your dislike of certain vegetables has less to do with taste and more to do with texture.

Seasonings!! This is a big one for me. Maybe you like lemon pepper?

It takes time for your taste buds and mind-set to adjust. Don't get into a power struggle with yourself. Small steps over time yield success in the long term.

Vitamins and PCOS

For most people, a balanced diet full of a variety of fruits, vegetables, and lean proteins provides all of the vitamins necessary to thrive; however, women with PCOS can benefit from vitamin supplements beyond a daily multivitamin. For example, birth control pills deplete vitamin B, folic acid, vitamin C, magnesium, and zinc. The medication metformin depletes vitamin B_{12}. The medication spironolactone can deplete folic acid, which is especially necessary to supporting healthy fetal development. This is why spironolactone is not recommended if you are thinking about becoming pregnant. Vitamin D deficiency is correlated with insulin resistance and fertility issues. Unfortunately, the cycle of vitamin D deficiency is self-perpetuating; since vitamin D is fat-soluble, excess fat in the body will absorb the vitamin D, resulting in lower vitamin D availability in the body.[4]

Often times, a vitamin B complex and a multivitamin can be helpful and resolve most issues related to vitamin deficiencies. I recommend taking your multivitamin at night to avoid any possible nausea and suggest taking your B vitamin in the morning, as it can provide an energy boost that might make it difficult to fall asleep.

As always, be sure to check with your doctor to make sure that supplements are right for you.

USING A DIET TRACKER:
IT'S MORE THAN COUNTING CALORIES

Most people think that using a diet tracker is tedious and restrictive. For women with PCOS, it can be an incredibly useful tool. Many believe that if they use a diet tracker, it's going to be too strict and controlling. I have actually found the opposite to be true. You can think of a diet tracker like a budget: once you know your calorie limit, you can decide how you want to "spend" your calories. It all comes down to balance. When you are out of your routine, the tracker gives you the flexibility to make the decisions that are right for you.

Unfortunately, women with PCOS cannot rely on commercial claims that a particular food is "healthy." What may be healthy for most women may be counterproductive for a woman with PCOS. For example, rice cakes and bananas are fine for women with no insulin issues but can spike blood sugar if you are insulin resistant. Tracking your food makes it easy to monitor nutritional values, macronutrients, and calories.

In addition, tracking your food can help create mindfulness around eating and help control cravings and binge eating. Give tracking your food an honest chance. It may feel overwhelming at first because you are not only tracking your food but also likely *giving much more energy to the foods you eat.* That's a lot of extra mental and emotional energy coming just from trying something. Remember the last time you started a job at a new office? Even if you know well how to do the actual work that you're doing, there's a lot of mental energy that goes into learning the quirks of the copy machine, the location of the light switches, and the passcodes to the new computer. After some time, all of that becomes automatic and less stressful. The same is true for tracking your food. At first, it takes more time than you think it should, but eventually it becomes easier. Using a diet-tracker app with a social-networking component can help you connect with other friends who use it. Some apps like My Fitness Pal will allow you to hide certain elements of your online profile—like your weight or the details of your food intake—from your friends list if you're not comfortable with that information being public.

Consistency in food tracking is essential. Less is more. When we are talking about a lifestyle change as a health strategy, it's far more effective to make modest changes that you can live with rather than make sweeping changes that will stress you out and burn you out in short order. Making changes to your diet means that you're making changes to your coping strategies, culture, habits, and more. It's important to make changes slowly and steadily to give yourself time to adjust.

If you eat it, track it. Don't cheat. You're not fooling anyone but yourself. Whether it's a cheating boyfriend or you cheating on your diet, I will tell you this: you deserve better. And there's no need to beat yourself up if you've fudged the numbers, but do look for the fear behind the behavior of altering the stats of what you eat.

Common trouble spots for maintaining a healthy diet include:

Too much, too soon—If you don't give your mind a chance to adjust to the new behavior you're taking on, the stress will cause you to abandon your plan. So take on one dietary change at a time, give it a few weeks to become a comfortable habit, and *then* move on to incorporating the next healthy change.

Change in routine—It's especially easy to fall off the wagon when traveling or around holidays. So when you know your schedule is going to be deviating from the norm, plan ahead: prepare healthy snacks to take along on trips, research online menus of the restaurants you're going to before you're hungry in order to identify the healthiest options you'll enjoy, and bring a satisfying, healthy dish to family functions centered on food.

Hydration—Often thirst is mistaken for hunger. So the next time you've recently eaten but you're still craving more food, first try drinking a tall glass of water and wait for about fifteen minutes. If the cravings persist, *then* consider eating again.

Internalizing all of these healthy-eating guidelines can feel overwhelming at first, and oftentimes people find it easier to not have to think through healthy-eating choices themselves but rely on an external rule or list. And so adhering to fad diets becomes attractive. While these popular eating plans may initially deplete less of your willpower, making it easier to reach the end of the day without a cookie binge, they also present their own mind-set and dietary stumbling blocks, so choose wisely.

Intermittent fasting—This type of diet requires fasting two days a week. There are several kinds of ways to do intermittent fasting. With 5:2 fasting, pick two nonconsecutive days to eat around 500 calories total.

The other days, eat as you normally would, paying attention, though, to your choices and portions. Proponents of this diet plan suggest that it produces weight loss and sensitizes insulin. If you have any issues with binge eating, anorexia, or any other eating disorder, intermittent fasting is likely not a safe option.

Ketogenic diet—This is a low- or no-carb, high-fat and -protein diet. When the body doesn't have carbohydrates for energy, it turns to fat stores in the liver, burning them instead. The ketogenic diet has been found to reduce free testosterone and contribute to weight loss; however, the results are not long-lasting. Most people regain the weight they lost on a ketogenic diet after a year. One reason for this is because it is a very strict diet, only creating change when followed to the letter. This makes it difficult to sustain in the long term. Also, once people attain the desired weight loss and resume eating normally, they tend to binge on foods that were previously forbidden on the ketogenic diet. There is also a concern that ketogenesis can cause muscle loss and extreme fatigue.[5]

Paleo diet—Adopting this diet means basically eating like a caveman would have: meat, vegetables, and fruit but absolutely no processed foods like bread, cereal, or candy. This eating pattern is beneficial because it eliminates many of the high-GI foods that can cause women with PCOS so much trouble; however, the Paleo diet also comes with the risk of eating too much protein and fat. If you choose to follow this diet, be sure to emphasize getting plenty of vegetables as well.[6]

Diet-in-a-box plans—I recommend that you avoid any diet plan that sells prepackaged meals. First, they are adjusted to be a good fit for someone with an average metabolism and insulin function. That's not you. Second, if they are prepackaged, they are loaded with salt, flavor enhancers, and preservatives. None of these things is good for your body. Third, if you stick with the program, then you don't learn anything about having a healthy relationship with nourishing food. I promise that the effort is worth the trouble. Choosing and, better yet, preparing your own meals means that you get maximum control over what you use to nourish your body. You can adjust any recipe to meet the nuances of your nutritional needs and allow for maximum flexibility in your life so that you don't miss out on anything.

What Happens if You Have an Off Day and You Completely Go Over in Calories?

That is not the end of the world. In fact, it's a learning opportunity, and it's completely normal. You can respond to that situation with gratitude and make adjustments.

It's ideal for women with PCOS to understand the finer points of a PCOS-friendly diet so that you can make those decisions with full understanding. I recommend that you try, adjust, and try again.

When my clients tell me they want to lose weight, I strongly recommend that they use a diet tracker. There are many free apps and programs online. I personally like My Fitness Pal, but I recommend that you play with a few and see which one you most prefer.

"How Do I Log This?"

If you plan on eating out, I strongly recommend that you plan your meal ahead. You might be surprised how many restaurants have their meals readily accessible on the fitness trackers. If you don't see it there, you may check out their website. This is especially important for women with PCOS, as most restaurants have added sugar in many of their foods. You might log a similar meal from another restaurant. As a last resort, you may have to log your meal piecemeal, ingredient by ingredient. For example, if you have a chicken salad from XYZ restaurant, you may log one chicken breast, 2 tablespoons of dressing, and 1 tablespoon of cheese. Focus on logging the higher-calorie, higher-fat items. Personally, I don't necessarily log lettuce, because it would be hard to blow your diet with that.

If you feel like using a diet tracker is too much trouble, consider another perspective: If you're overweight and have PCOS, you're likely spending a lot of time and emotional energy worrying about your weight and health issues. Imagine what it would be like if you looked forward to going shopping, looked forward to that next big social event, and in general went through your daily life loving the way your body looked and felt. Once you get the hang of it, tracking really doesn't take much time out of your day.

Some people plan their meals out at the beginning of the day, pretracking everything, and then follow that plan. Others log as they go. I suggest you try both approaches to see what works for you. If you can help it, try not to leave all of your diet tracking until the end of the day; it's too easy to forget what you actually ate or to decide not to do it at all when faced with logging breakfast, lunch, dinner, and snacks when you're exhausted.

Feeling the urge to hit the fast food restaurant on the way home? Pull over and log it in your diet tracker first. Chances are, when you see the hard caloric and macronutrient evidence of what you're craving, the desire to actually eat it will diminish. Also, an average craving lasts only fifteen minutes, so by slowing down to log your potential meal, you're giving yourself time to let the craving pass.

Often clients ask me, *Why should I use a diet tracker? Can't I just eat healthily?* The bottom line is that too few of us have properly internalized what healthy portion sizes truly are, and it's far too easy to blow your calorie budget in one poorly planned meal even after a full day at the gym. And if you're overweight, it might take time to adjust your body to a new definition of healthy eating and sufficient portion sizes. It's okay to take your time with this process and drop your calorie goals slowly. Some diet gurus suggest that if we center ourselves and listen to our bodies, then we will naturally know what and how much to eat. In this day and age, I respectfully disagree. While it would be lovely to have time to meditate or journal several times a day, I know very few women who have that luxury. I suggest that by logging your food and exercise, you simplify that process of self-discovery and set yourself up for measurable success.

"Will I Have to Track My Food Forever?"

Probably. PCOS is a lifelong syndrome. To successfully manage it for the rest of your life, you cannot take a set-it-and-forget-it approach. It's to be expected that your life will evolve over time, with plenty of ups and downs along the way—not only physically but also emotionally. The same way that someone with diabetes must forever monitor their blood sugar, you will do well to log your food. Using the right tools can help make your efforts more effective and efficient so that you stay focused no matter what. Remember that a diet tracker is not the boss of you, nor is it there to judge. It is simply a tool. You choose how you want to use it.

It's important to remember that learning to use a diet- and fitness-tracking app takes practice. You're going to have easy days and harder days. This is really where seeing a registered dietitian, working with a healthy-eating support group, or pursuing another type of coaching can be useful (more on professional support in chapter 11). Remember, you're not talking about a short-term adjustment but a lifestyle change.

HYDRATION

One often-overlooked trigger for overeating is dehydration. Ever wonder why your cravings are worse in the afternoon or evening? It could be due to dehydration. When you feel a craving coming on, it's important to not rush to the closest bag of chips but slow the process down so that you can identify what's really going on with your body. You may have heard that you need to drink eight glasses of water per day; however, this is simply an easily remembered amount that is generally enough for most women. While the exact measurement of ideal intake is hotly debated, the bottom line is that most people aren't getting nearly enough water and are living life chronically dehydrated. Water is an essential component of every bodily process and can even affect mood. Ensuring an adequate amount of water can alleviate many symptoms often erroneously attributed to something else—like hunger.

The body begins sending out signals of dehydration long before we are in danger. Chronic dehydration can make you feel fatigued, which makes getting enough exercise difficult. It can also lower your mood. Tryptophan is a precursor of serotonin, the "feel-good" neurotransmitter. Chronic dehydration limits the ability of tryptophan to get into your brain. The liver also pulls tryptophan to help out when the body is dehydrated, which further decreases its availability. If you are chronically dehydrated and suffer from depression, drinking more water may not be a cure-all, but it will certainly fill a gap that needs to be filled.

Dehydration doesn't necessarily cause anxiety, but it can cause symptoms that we mistake for anxiety, such as a rapid heart rate and dizziness. Often it is these physical symptoms that can trigger a panic attack, so staying hydrated is an important prevention strategy if you struggle with anxiety.

Physical signs of mild to moderate dehydration include headache, dry mouth, thirst, fatigue, and dizziness. Signs of severe dehydration include seizure, amber-colored urine, poor skin elasticity, and rapid heart rate. If you take the medication spironolactone, it is especially important that you get enough water, as the medication acts as a diuretic, pulling water from your body.

Some tips to staying hydrated include:

Sipping water throughout the day—Keeping a water bottle close will make it more likely you'll adequately hydrate.

Limiting coffee, alcohol, and energy drinks—They have a diuretic effect.

Ditching the soda—Whether the regular or diet kind, sodas with caffeine can dehydrate you. Even the caffeine-free kind is filled with unhealthy chemicals.

Drinking more water, herbal tea, and sparkling water—Juice isn't a good option because of the sugar content.

Adding frozen fruit to your water—This adds a flavor boost and is a nice changeup from ice cubes.

Being especially aware of times when you're out of your routine—Throwing off your routine, such as when traveling, can result in dehydration.

Setting reminders—Set a couple of timed alarms on your smartphone, especially if there's a time of day when you tend to forget to drink enough water.

Connecting habits—Mentally link your new water-drinking habit to other habits that are already established, like drinking a tall glass of water while waiting for your morning coffee to brew or sipping from a water bottle while on your way to and from work.

BARIATRIC SURGERY

One option for weight loss is bariatric surgery. There are many different types of this surgical procedure, and if you are considering it, it's important to talk with your health-care provider about the best option for you. Whatever the type, bariatric surgery is a surgical intervention that limits the volume of food that can be ingested at any one time. Nutritional availability can also be impacted by bariatric surgery, as digestion time is impacted by the fat and protein content in foods, which can in turn impact the rate at which the body can absorb nutrients. In essence, bariatric surgery is meant to resolve a mind-set issue, and it is not for everyone. As we know, the average food craving lasts for about fifteen minutes. This means that for most people, a combination of mind-set work, emotional support, and medical intervention are sufficient to learning how to make healthy, sustainable eating choices; however, when the issue around food is too significant and all other options have been exhausted, then bariatric surgery might be a last resort. That does not mean that choosing bariatric surgery is indicative of weakness or brokenness, for even the bariatric-surgical patient must still do the mind-set work and embrace all of the lifestyle strategies. If healthy lifestyle changes aren't made, then the results of the surgery will not be successful, since there are ways to "cheat" the surgery, and those modifications are extremely dangerous. Bariatric surgery is simply a way to help a person to slow down the process of feeling a craving and the response to it so that there is time for an awareness to develop. Bariatric surgery serves as a definitive mark, not only for the patient but also for the family, that a lifestyle change is happening. This can cause significant upset for all involved. In fact, chance of divorce skyrockets following bariatric surgery. The question then becomes *Will bariatric surgery improve PCOS?* The answer is yes . . . and no. In one sense, undergoing bariatric surgery limits the amount of food you eat, which might help with insulin resistance; however, you still must make choices about the *macros* in what you are eating. The surgery can't make that choice for you. But certainly significant weight loss through bariatric surgery can help get PCOS symptoms under control, reduce cardiovascular limitations, and help make exercise more comfortable.

DIET AS SELF-CARE

One of the kindest things you can do for yourself is to consistently eat healthy foods. By choosing your nutrition, you are choosing one powerful way of nurturing yourself. Preparing meals for yourself instead of tolerating prepackaged meals will help you feel vibrant, centered, and cared for. It becomes so comforting that when you don't have healthy meals, you are left feeling insecure and out of balance. If that happens, you can start over with a clean slate and recommit to treating yourself with love, one meal at a time.

JOURNALING QUESTIONS

1. What can healthy eating do for me?
2. What are the "special occasions" when it's okay to splurge on less healthy food?
3. Where are my diet trouble spots?
4. Why haven't I made changes in my eating habits before now?

3

❖ ❖

Exercise for Women with PCOS

Exercise is the single most misunderstood and undervalued part of recovery from PCOS. In fact, consistent exercise goes beyond burning calories and can actually have a powerful therapeutic effect on almost every aspect of PCOS. Some women are so flatly opposed to the idea of exercise that they would prefer to limit calories rather than exercise. This is a mistake, as the benefits of exercise go beyond calorie burn. *When it comes to long-term health, you get back what you give.* You will get out of exercise exactly what you put in. This sort of clarity gives you the opportunity to stress less and create balance in your life.

The question, very often, is *Where do I even start?*

Start where you are, not where you think you should be. Change should be slow—so slow you wonder if it's working but you feel giddy over how easy it feels. That second part is crucial. Most women who have PCOS have spent years fighting with their bodies. If asked, they can give a detailed list of what their bodies can't do. The first goal of exercise is to redefine that perspective. Take the list of what your body can't do and toss it out of the window. Even if the list seems accurate, it's not helping in the least, and it's time to release the inner critic that is supporting it. The time has come to make a list of what your body can do, and exercise is the place to start.

Start simply. You can always increase the intensity later on, but if you do too much too soon, you'll quickly burn out or, worse, injure yourself. When starting an exercise routine, stop before feeling fatigued. You're looking for that motivational sweet spot that will serve you well when it comes to making exercise a daily part of life.

Your goal isn't to lose weight—it's to gain health. The reality is that once you reach your goal weight, you still have to keep going with your wellness activities. Start the way you mean to go on—not in intensity but in the way you want to feel about exercise. The definition of what comprises ideal exercise will naturally vary from one person to the next; however, there are guidelines that will transform exercise into lasting lifestyle change.

Current research indicates that it takes "vigorous" exercise to reverse insulin resistance, which usually does one of two things: (1) you will feel overwhelmed and do nothing, or (2) you will go to the gym with the intention of pushing yourself to the physical limit every day. While saying yes to an over-the-top exercise program may seem logical, it is a mistake if your goal is consistency. Many women who have PCOS are frustrated and angry with their bodies. The urge to *force* exercise and *control* diet seems to be the only way forward, but that only ever works in the short term. PCOS is a chronic condition, which means you need to create a manageable, long-term solution. Exercising to the point of pain is the fastest way to destroy your motivation. Instead, the solution is to respond to this call to action with respect and gratitude for what your body gives you.

CALL A TRUCE WITH YOUR BODY

It will be no fun to connect with your body the way you do when you're exercising if you are at war with it. Make a list of the things you love about your body.

In order to protect long-term motivation, begin with an open, curious mind-set, and resist the urge to judge your starting point. If walking for ten minutes is a challenge, that's okay. Start there. *Your motivation is only as strong as it is on your worst day*, so if a ten-minute walk is what you can do on your worst day, then that's fine. Exercise every day unless you are sick or injured. Exercise should challenge your body but should never hurt. Our bodies were designed to move and feel good. This is actually what motivates the vast majority of our thoughts and actions in every aspect of life.

WHAT'S THE BEST EXERCISE?

I'm often asked what the best exercise is for weight loss. *The bottom line is that the best exercise is the one you'll actually do.* The goal is to determine what will work with your lifestyle, time availability, and personal preference. It does not matter whether an exercise is the latest, greatest, and most efficient; if you don't enjoy it, then you won't stick with it. Almost any exercise can be modified to fit your needs and abilities.

Attempting an exercise that you don't enjoy means that you have to go through an extra step to achieve your goal. It is that extra step of having to talk yourself into doing an exercise you don't enjoy that creates the motivation gap.

The solution is to pick an exercise that you can easily adjust over time. Your exercise of choice should be accessible no matter what. Remember that motivation gap I mentioned? There are few things more motivation killing than having to drive across town in rush-hour traffic to a gym where you have to wait to use a certain machine. Identify the gaps in your motivation. What is keeping you from reaching your daily goals?

If you're too scared, intimidated, or shy to work out, remember that everyone started somewhere. You might have seen a case of body shaming come across your newsfeed, but those are few and far between. What impresses the already-fit crowd is your commitment to being consistent in your efforts.

CARDIO

I highly recommend walking and/or running as your cardio exercise, because it is simple and portable and can be easily adjusted from one day to the next. Many people ask about couch-to-5k programs as go-to exercise plans; I'd say they're great *if* you use them correctly.

Consider signing up for a couch-to-5k program. These programs—often available as apps—are designed to get even the worst kind of couch potato fit enough to run a 5k after a specified course of training. The program intensity starts low and helps users gradually build up stamina and time running. However, the couch-to-5k apps don't know you. They don't know whether you slept well, had an argument with your spouse, or are dehydrated. They are also not the boss of you. You are the boss of you. Here's the secret to successfully using a couch-to-5k app: do it *every* day, and *repeat days as necessary*. If you try a day that feels like it's too much of a jump in intensity, then repeat the previous day's workout. Stay there for a few days until it feels better, and then try going on to the next day's workout. Not all apps give you the option to do this, so be sure to check out the program features before deciding on one version or another. I like the Zen Labs' couch-to-5k app, but the options are essentially endless.

If walking or running isn't your thing, that's okay. The principle is the same: find an exercise that you can do every day, anywhere, that feels good at your starting point, gets your heart rate up, and can be scaled to your current fitness level.

One caveat about cardio: *don't overdo it*. The last thing you want is to overstress your body, which will only result in muscle loss and *increased* insulin resistance. The ideal amount of exercise time is from thirty to sixty minutes. Anything beyond that and you risk muscle loss, injury, or burnout.

> **TIP:** If you don't feel like exercising one day, I strongly encourage you to use the *ten-minute rule*: Unless you are sick or injured, go do your cardio for at least ten minutes. If you feel like continuing, great! If you still want to stop after ten minutes, that's okay. The point is that you respect yourself enough to try and then to stop when you need to. I encourage you to try this. It's a powerful step and can be a thrill that spills over into other areas of your life where you have to put effort in *and* set limits.

WHAT ABOUT WEIGHT LIFTING?

Women who have PCOS should definitely add weight lifting to their exercise plan. Here's why:

Extra muscle helps control and reduce insulin resistance.
Muscle supports the body in everyday life.
Weight training boosts metabolism for a greater calorie burn throughout the day.
And it can improve balance.

You may be concerned about putting on too much muscle, but not to worry. Even with the additional testosterone that is common for women with PCOS, it is impossible to achieve a bodybuilder physique unless you are deliberately working hard to do so. And doing so requires *hours* of specialized training in the gym.

MAINTAIN YOUR MOTIVATION TO DO HOME WORKOUTS

It's hard to beat the convenience of home workouts, but special care must be given to maintaining motivation. It's helpful to work out at the same time each day. This helps you create a routine and prioritize your time rather than making exercise an afterthought to fit in as you have time.

Release the "should," and do what speaks to you. If you know you should stretch every day but don't really enjoy it, then do something that you do enjoy, like pull-ups or squats. Use the ten-minute rule.

Very often it's hard to transition from home life to exercise time. Try to work out in a place that is dedicated just to your exercise. While it may be tempting to throw down a yoga mat in any room of the house, having a dedicated space helps you maintain your focus. Create a ritual for setting the stage for exercise. This might be lighting a candle, opening up the windows, or something else that serves as a visual reminder that this time is separate from your other daily tasks. I can guarantee you that every gym has a protocol for whatever they consider ideal lighting, temperature, and music. You can do the same thing at home. Make it something simple but significant. Listen to music to help your mind switch gears and get focused. This is a great way to elevate your mood so that you can get started with exercise.

Exercise at the same time every day so that it becomes your routine. This also helps family and friends know what to expect. Be patient but firm with family members and friends. There might be an adjustment period with them, especially if they are used to you being available any time.

Keep a pad of paper and a pen by your workout area. Jot down whatever to-dos that come to mind so you don't feel compelled to run off and do them right then. You can also use another sheet to record your exercise accomplishments for the day so you can track progress over time.

HOW TO SET EXERCISE GOALS

The best way to set your exercise goals is to decide on your ultimate fitness goal and get crystal clear on what that entails. While it's okay to have a weight-loss goal, it's important to explore your feelings about using your body in a healthy way. Set realistic, measurable health goals for yourself. People are always saying to aim high, but for the majority of people trying to get healthier, that is terrible advice. While professional athletes may be adept at extreme choices that support making a living with their skills and passion, it's okay for you to set a more modest progression toward your goals.

Once you have clarified your ultimate fitness goal, reverse engineer it. Work backward from that goal until you are where you are now, fitness-wise. For example, if you have set a goal to run a 5k, don't go out and see how far you can push yourself on day one. Instead, set a goal—continuously running for 3.1 miles—and plan backward—continuously running for two miles, running for one mile, running for ten minutes, and so on—until you get to your current athletic capability. Be honest and kind to yourself, and decide what feels good. For example, does walking a mile feel like something you could do every day? If the answer is yes, then draw a map from your goal (running a 5k) back to where you are right now. The biggest mistake is to push for too much too fast. That only creates stress, which is not good for a woman with PCOS. Instead, set daily microgoals that are attainable and are working in the direction of your ultimate fitness goal. Can you do more than you planned to that day? Sure! You'll certainly have your share of motivated, energetic days. Keep in mind though that your body is not a machine, so it's okay on those tougher days to fall back to the ten-minute rule as a placeholder while you attend to any emotional, physical, and mental resistance that may be keeping you from your workout.

Be sure to celebrate the achievement of each and every goal. Meeting a daily goal matters and is reason to smile!

HOW TO MAKE EXERCISE PART OF YOUR ROUTINE

Most people take an all-or-nothing approach to exercise. We do this because our minds are designed to categorize, to set things into compact, orderly groups. The reality for most people is that life is entirely too complicated.

Between family responsibilities, that looming deadline at work, and the fact that maybe you didn't get enough sleep last night, there is tremendous variation in the way your body and mind can feel from day to day. You are not a machine. Exercise isn't a set-it-and-forget-it endeavor. Instead, allow for variation within the routine. Invite the exercise to meet you where you are. Some days you might want to do some sprints; other days you might want a casual stroll through the local botanical garden.

TIP: Don't be afraid of terms like *sprints* or *high-intensity interval training*. HIIT, as it's known, is a popular option for cardio, but it is often misunderstood. Designed to enhance fitness and fat loss, HIIT alternates intervals of high-intensity and low-intensity exercise. By definition, HIIT is exercising to increase your heart rate up to between 70 and 90 percent of your maximum heart rate, followed by a rest period, which brings your heart rate back down to between 60 and 65 percent, and then repeating cycles of high intensity and rest for the duration of the established workout time. If you enjoy more variety over monotonous walking or running at the same pace, HIIT might be an option to explore. There are plenty of apps to help you keep track of your time between intervals. You define what high intensity means for you. No need to run sprints up stairs if you're not ready for it. The point is to get your heart rate up in regular intervals within the workout. You don't want to do something so far outside of your comfort zone that it is detrimental to your health. "High intensity" may mean running as fast as you can, but it may also mean swinging your arms a bit faster as you walk on the treadmill. Listen to your body, and adjust each activity to meet you where you are right now.

YOU ARE WHAT YOU REPEATEDLY DO

People often wonder whether they should work out every day or take a rest day. While most exercise plans try to woo you with promises of results from a mere three days a week of exercise, buying in would be a mistake in terms of motivation. Motivation and habit work very closely with one another, so it pays to do some kind of exercise every day. Decrease the intensity if you need to; keep it fresh by exercising in different locations if that's important to you. Your body is designed to move, so exercising every day is ideal. That said, rest days aren't all bad; you just have to do them right. For example, you might want to schedule a rest day on the weekend so that you can focus on time with family. The mistake comes when you give yourself a wild-card rest day, because what will happen is that one random rest day turns into two rest days, and then pretty soon you're not working out at all.

If you typically exercise outside, you want to establish a plan B. It doesn't have to be a perfectly matched replacement, but it does have to be ready to use. For example, don't think of jumping rope as your rainy-day plan unless you actually own a jump rope. Plan ahead so that doing the alternative is uncomplicated.

The best exercise is the one that requires the least amount of effort to get started. You have to be honest with yourself about any roadblocks when deciding on an exercise program. Working out at home is a fantastic alternative to the gym, but many people struggle with getting into the exercise mind-set. It's hard to switch gears. Invariably, other responsibilities creep in and take the joy and effectiveness from your exercise time—the time when you're supposed to be doing the most self-care.

WHAT COUNTS AS EXERCISE

We all have different levels of activity. This can vary based on your job, your family life, your hobbies, or even your personality. When you're counting exercise, your normal activity level should not count toward your exercise goals. Only count those things like cardio and weight-training activities as exercise. Logging the walk from the parking lot into the grocery store is simply an opportunity to be grateful to use your body. The only exception to this rule is if you have been living an extremely sedentary lifestyle and this type of movement is entirely new. In that case, celebrate each step.

THAT FIRST WEEK

Like learning the strategies of a new diet plan, extra mental effort is required when beginning a new exercise routine: the mind has to work harder at first, figuring out how to adjust the machines, how to transition from one move to the next, or how to figure out which is the right setting on the workout app you're using. There is a tremendous amount of mental energy that may temporarily take away from the flow and enjoyment of exercise, but know that it is only temporary. Start with shorter workouts and stick with them, and you will find that exercise is a way to feel better, stronger, and more relaxed every time you do it.

WORKING AROUND HEALTH ISSUES AND INJURIES

If you suffer from chronic pain or conditions such as bad knees or arthritis, you still don't have a valid excuse not to exercise! There are always modifications. I highly suggest performing YouTube and other Google searches for creative exercise ideas and examples. That said, never do anything that could potentially hurt you; nurturing your body is top priority.

Bottom line: start where you are. After my second child was born, I felt like running was useless for me because I could "only" run for twenty seconds at a time. It turns out there is no "only." I learned that twenty seconds is better than zero seconds and that walking is a valuable and valid exercise.

Exercise should make you feel challenged, excited, and invigorated. The most important factor for success is not intensity but consistency. Exercise *every day*.

No one is judging your starting point. *Except maybe you, so be nice.*

WHO DO YOU THINK YOU ARE? AN ATHLETE

When I'm talking to a client and refer to her as an athlete, she very often will shrink back and laugh nervously or roll her eyes and tell me that she is far from being an athlete. The reality is that we all are athletes. The limiting factor is not in our physical ability; rather, it is our mind. Examine your definition of an athlete. An athlete is a person who takes consistent focused action to improve her physical ability. It may be in a group sport, or it may be an individual pursuit like running. What do you think about yourself? How do you think about yourself? This is a tough one for women with PCOS—especially if you've come to believe that your body is broken or defective in some way. As women with PCOS, we have a metabolic issue, but our bodies are far from broken. Exercise is your daily reminder that your body is strong and capable. Repeating that message on a daily basis will help you connect with that confidence in other parts of your life and elevate your sense of accomplishment and self-worth. Elevating your self-worth makes it infinitely easier to justify taking precious time out of your day for exercise. If you have always reserved the title of "athlete" for only the elite, then I encourage you to broaden that perspective.

Consider a few excellent reasons to exercise—ones that have nothing to do with fitness:

Exercise reduces stress hormones—Cortisol is the most widely known stress hormone. Did you know that it is tied to weight gain and inflammation? A daily workout can ease stress and reduce cortisol, but be sure that the exercise isn't so vigorous that it creates more stress! If possible, women with PCOS should exercise in the morning when cortisol levels are highest.

Exercise reduces anxiety—Everyone experiences anxiety from time to time, and some cope with it daily. Consistent exercise can reduce anxiety. Thirty minutes of cardio per day is best, but even a ten-minute walk outside can help take the edge off anxiety. This doesn't have to be an intense sweat session.

Exercise elevates mood—Just like anxiety, feeling down in the dumps is a part of life. Depression is often described as anger turned inward. While exercise likely won't cure major depressive disorder, it certainly won't hurt. For people with normal fluctuations in mood, it's helpful to know that exercise is a solution that is readily available and effective. (More on depression in chapter 6.)

Exercise improves creativity and flow—You don't have to be an artist to benefit from improved creativity. Creative problem solving can help with everyday challenges.

Exercise contributes to body confidence—Confidence is attractive. Consistent exercise improves strength, tone, coordination, and balance. Noticing your body change and improve over time will give you a sense of accomplishment that spreads to every area of your life.

Morning exercise positively impacts your entire day—Exercising first thing sets the tone for healthy choices throughout the day.

Exercise is excellent self-care—If you struggle to put yourself on top of your priority list, you're not alone. If you're angry with your body for what it can't do, it's hard to consider making time to care for it. It's time to call a truce and get on a healthy track.

Exercise improves your relationships—One of the most powerful examples you can give someone is treating yourself the way you want to be treated. Up-level your relationships with daily exercise.

Exercise improves your sleep—A daily exercise routine helps regulate sleep cycles. It eases stress, quiets the mind, and relaxes the body, which in turn can improve sleep. Regular sleep reduces food cravings too, so you can more easily stay on track with your diet.

EVALUATING YOUR EXERCISE GOALS AND ACCOMPLISHMENTS

After a few weeks of consistent exercise, take a look at your progress. What has changed? How far have you come? No change is insignificant. Remember, you only have to lose around 5–10 percent of your body weight to experience dramatic improvements in health, including insulin sensitivity and lowered testosterone levels.

When you evaluate your exercise plan, be sure to check in with both your body *and your mind*. Pain during or after your workout is a warning. If your workout was strenuous to the point that afterward you couldn't carry out your normal daily activities without being in pain, scale back the intensity—but keep doing something every day. A brisk walk is often enough to warm up and loosen your muscles so that you are more comfortable throughout the rest of your day. If the exercise felt easy, consider stepping it up a bit—but not too much! It's okay to take a week or so to find your ideal starting point. Consider tracking your exercise to make it easier to evaluate changes. Being able to look back on your progress can help you overcome insecurity and doubt. Tracking your progress in exercise is a lot like tracking your weight loss: you are looking for general trends, not perfectly linear progress.

PAIN VERSUS DISCOMFORT

Have you ever heard these?

"No pain, no gain."
"Sweat is weakness leaving the body."
"Get whipped into shape!"

These popular sayings are catchy, and perhaps sound cool, but for most people they are motivation killers. It's time to ditch the myth that you will benefit from painful exercise. When done correctly (with self-respect and consistency), exercise can be a powerful tool to ease the pervasive effects of PCOS.

Exercise should not hurt. Some fitness gurus will tell you that enduring pain is fine, even helpful, as long as you don't injure yourself. To me, this borders on hazing—like we have seen on college campuses. You shouldn't have to grit your teeth just to push through exercise. Our minds are designed to avoid pain. If you take on an exercise program that elicits pain, I can guarantee that your mind will work hard to keep you from continuing it. Exercise should feel challenging and invigorating.

It's important to make the distinction between pain and discomfort. Pain is a negative feeling, and our minds naturally avoid it. It is a warning sign to our bodies that injury is highly possible. However, mild discomfort is a normal and acceptable part of exercise. The trick is to know the difference and respect your body's needs and limits. You shouldn't feel bullied by personal trainers or your inner critic! We don't exercise for a short-term goal. As women with PCOS, *we exercise to redefine our relationship with our body.* If you struggle with the boundary between pain and discomfort or are prone to self-injurious behavior, always err on the side of caution.

Discomfort during exercise can also come in the form of emotional discomfort. It is not uncommon for strong feelings to come up during exercise. Exercise brings up a lot of thoughts and emotional energy that we have tended to tamp down throughout the rest of our day. Negative thoughts are as draining as carrying around a backpack full of lead. To maximize your energy, acknowledge the negative thoughts as they come up, and then release them as you exercise and keep going. Emotional discomfort rising to the surface of your awareness happens for a few reasons: Your day-to-day life might be so busy that negative feelings don't have a chance to be acknowledged otherwise. Or perhaps it could be that you're releasing some emotional stress that was long held in your body. In order to maintain your motivation in the face of these thoughts and feelings, I recommend you acknowledge them and, to the degree you are able, release them while you continue exercise. Keep your thoughts positive. Let your body have a turn to be front and center for a bit. If you have found journaling helpful, then journal about it at some point, or perhaps talk to someone you trust—a friend or counselor—to work through any issues that cause extreme upset or continue to come up. Try shifting your focus to your body during exercise: notice the way your legs feel, feel the air go in and out of your lungs, clench your hands into fists and slowly release—whatever it takes to bring awareness into your body.

CARDIO FOR MINDFULNESS

Running is part of my daily routine. I trust my body that I can comfortably run three to five miles. I can tell you, though, that sometimes the first half mile is uncomfortable. Maybe I'm stiff from sleeping funny, or maybe my body isn't warmed up yet. I have learned to tolerate a bit of discomfort that I trust will give way to an incredible feeling of satisfaction at the end of the run. On occasion, my body has given me signals that the run isn't going to happen. For example, a time or two I have gotten a stitch in my side that I simply couldn't work through. So I cut my run short. No big deal. I spent the walk home thinking about what might have caused it without taking a blaming, negative tone with myself. It was more of a mildly curious voice: "Hmmm . . . did I drink enough water yesterday?" On occasion, during my runs I've had some emotions come up that were very powerful. I trusted that I could work through them later in the day but that the best thing for me was to nurture my body with this run.

How do you get comfortable with the *discomfort* of exercise? Start simply. Build slowly. If you push too hard and too fast, you will feel pain, which might mentally reinforce the belief that you can't exercise. When it comes to long-term motivation, creating emotional stamina and confidence are just as important as developing physical stamina.

ROADBLOCKS TO EXERCISE

"It Won't Work"

If you're worried that your exercise routine won't produce results, you're likely setting goals that are either too widely spaced or only of one type. There are many different ways to measure progress, and not all of them have to do with jean size or the number on the scale. This is especially true for women with PCOS. Expand your measures of success to include increased energy and confidence and reduced mood swings or blood pressure. There may be times when you see progress in some areas that have little to do with weight, but it still counts as working on other areas of your health and well-being, and these goals are no less important.

When you're thinking about goals and measures of success, be sure that you don't compare yourself to other women. Everyone has different responsibilities, strengths, and passions. It's okay to not do the fitness-model or professional-athlete routine. Every exercise that you do should feel good. You should feel pumped and excited about your next session.

"It Won't Be Enough"

There are a lot of factors that come together to produce change. Fitness isn't all or nothing. You can be fit and healthy yet still have potential for improvement. It takes very little exercise to create discernable change; the key is to do it *consistently* and in conjunction with other healthy lifestyle habits—like sufficient sleep, stress management, and good hydration.

"I Don't Have Enough Energy"

While fatigue is a real issue for women with PCOS, it's very hard to distinguish mental fatigue from physical fatigue. Assuming you aren't sick or have a medical reason why you should not exercise, try exercising for ten minutes before deciding whether are too tired. A depressed mood can be confused with physical fatigue. A ten-minute workout is often enough to boost your mood and actually give you more energy overall. Consistent exercise, especially when done earlier in the day, has been shown to improve sleep, which can also boost your energy levels.

"I'm Too Busy"

When a client tells me this, we talk about her schedule and her list of priorities. Very often, she has put herself at the bottom of a long list of must-dos. Everyone has different responsibilities, strengths, and passions. Where are you in your list of priorities? It's not about finding time; it's about making time. When you become a priority, the time to take care of yourself will be there. While I'm not a huge fan of training like a top athlete, there is one main takeaway from their approach: be unwavering in your commitment to consistency! You don't have to train for hours a day; however, I want every exercise that you do to feel good so that you are pumped and excited to do the next one. Thirty minutes of consistent work every day can be truly life changing.

"I'll Look Foolish"/"People Will Stare at Me"

This excuse breaks my heart, mostly because I've been there and I know what a very real fear this can be, especially for women with PCOS as we are more prone to social anxiety. Despite the horror stories you may have seen on social media, there are droves of gym-goers who are more than happy to help you figure out the equipment and thrilled to watch you crush your goals with consistent and focused exercise.

EQUIPMENT: WHAT'S NECESSARY, WHAT'S FUN, AND WHAT'S A TOTAL SHAM

If you're like many women, you set an exercise goal and buy some expensive piece of exercise equipment associated with that goal. What happens, more often than not, is that this exercise equipment becomes a glorified clothing rack. When it comes to equipment, less is usually more.

Children have more fun and exhibit heightened creative play with fewer toys. The same can be said for minimal exercise equipment. When you're getting started, it's helpful to limit your purchases to just the necessities so that you keep your motivation internally focused and avoid depending on a piece of equipment to motivate you.

What's Necessary

Necessary equipment provides safety and enough comfort so that the exercise you're doing can feel good. Examples of necessary equipment might be well-fitting shoes for walking or running. The most efficient way to find well-fitting shoes is to visit a shoe store that specializes in walking or running shoes. They will evaluate your stride and the way your foot falls as you walk and then give you options for shoes that will support and balance your stride. If you're feeling like you're not "enough" of an athlete to warrant proper footwear, I encourage you to reconsider. I've never heard of a single instance of negativity with these sorts of stores. The truth is that walkers and runners come in all shapes and sizes. This is especially important if you have joint pain. Many of my clients have experienced joint pain in their hips and knees that resolved once they started wearing well-fitting shoes.

Another bit of necessary equipment is a supportive sports bra. If you are larger-chested, this can be easier said than done, but it is well worth the effort. Keep in mind, not all double-Ds are created equal, so a sports bra that works for one woman might not work for another. Keep trying until you find what works for you. It will up-level your cardio experience and help you feel freer in your workouts.

Equipment for modifications is also necessary. For example, if you enjoy yoga but struggle with flexibility, a yoga block is necessary. Sure, you can use furniture or books, but an actual yoga block removes the extra mental energy of trying out modifications.

What's Fun

Wearable fitness trackers are all the rage these days but are not necessary. That said, many women enjoy having the extra data that comes from a wearable device. Their benefit is that you can get feedback that supports your overall wellness. For example, information on heart rate gives valuable information to help with stress management. You can also get useful information on sleep habits and sleep quality. It's a fun way to get feedback on the things that you will likely learn to feel intuitively.

As for secondary exercise equipment, I recommend that you have a go-to cardio exercise, and if you want to do more, then by all means make sure you have the equipment you need. For example, if you usually walk but enjoy rollerblading, then make sure you have the proper-fitting roller-blades and helmet and pads necessary to keeping it safe and fun.

What's a Total Sham

In my opinion, a large piece of equipment that works only one part of the body is absolutely unnecessary. Unless you have unlimited space and money for the investment, these types of machines typically become more of a nuisance in your home than a well-used piece of equipment.

Also, equipment that is marketed to give you "effortless results" is also not helpful. If it sounds too good to be true, it probably is. There should be an exciting, pleasant challenge associated with exercise. Our bodies are meant to be used! No need to make it unnoticeable. The way you define that challenge is what makes you unique. What you do today impacts your tomorrow, and your choices today are relevant to the story you are creating. Make them awesome.

JOURNAL QUESTIONS

1. What's your ideal exercise routine?
2. What beliefs about exercise have been holding you back?
3. How do you want to feel before, during, and after exercise?
4. What are the most important benefits of exercise for you?
5. What do you perceive the obstacles to exercise are for you? How might you overcome them?

4

Sleep

An Essential Healing Technique

When busy people run out of time to accomplish everything they think they must accomplish in their day, they often decide to stay up late or wake up early to fit everything in. They borrow time from their sleep—or, more precisely, they steal sleep from themselves. However, sleep is more than a convenient comfort. It's an essential component of a healthy lifestyle. It is widely known that the human mind and body require between seven and eight hours of sleep per night to function at its best. An occasional lost hour of sleep might not have a huge effect, but chronic sleep deprivation can be devastating to your health.

We tend to think of getting healthy as something we do, but when it comes to sleep, it is something we allow. Our bodies do amazing things while we sleep that are essential for mental and physical health. The effort is in setting boundaries and managing our internal dialogue in the process so that we get a sufficient amount of sleep on a consistent schedule.

Sleep is often seen as a nonessential task, and we feel selfish for taking more than the bare minimum. We commonly make empty promises to ourselves that we will "make it up" on the weekends. That doesn't actually work; it only causes frustration and stress when the sleep you thought you would get is interrupted. Most women fear that not checking everything off the list before going to bed is a sign of failure or a lack of drive. This need to live up to a superwoman image is the enemy of sleep. You can say no and still be a good person.

Just because the health implications of sleep deprivation might not be immediate doesn't mean they are not there. Many women play a dangerous game of sleep limbo: How low can you go before you collapse? Most women strike this deal so seamlessly that it is barely noticeable, even to them, but it's important to give the deficit ample consideration. The purpose of getting insight in this problem isn't to lay blame on anyone or anything. The purpose is to give you more information to work with so that you prioritize your list of must-dos. The fact is that you have to take care of yourself first. In an airplane, you put the oxygen mask on yourself before helping others. Being at your best—being healthy, alert, and energetic—is the ideal way to help others. You can't get that way by being chronically sleep-deprived. When you get enough sleep, you are more likely to plow through your to-do list in a timely fashion and feel good doing it.

Sometimes lost hours of sleep are unavoidable. And that's okay. It's when the quick fix becomes a habit that your health begins to suffer. So instead of taking time from your sleep to meet your obligations, look for other ways to find time in your day. Try to consolidate tasks for those things that don't require your full attention. For example, add folding your laundry to your TV time. Say no to taking on additional responsibilities when you can, and release the need to be everything to everyone. You probably can't do everything on your (or their) list, and the truth is, that's okay. Give yourself permission to let go of whatever you can and to make yourself a priority. Managing a chronic illness requires that you do just that: manage it. As a woman with PCOS, getting good sleep is a nonnegotiable part of that plan. *Inadequate sleep will undermine all of your other health efforts.*

BENEFITS FOR MIND AND BODY

Sleep is when our bodies do most of their healing. This is certainly true for the cardiovascular system. Chronic sleep deprivation is linked to higher rates of stroke, high blood pressure, and heart disease.[1]

Another hit to heart health is the increased risk in obesity among the sleep-deprived. Lack of sleep increases blood sugar and insulin. Elevated blood sugar is related to a hardening of the arteries and the development of type 2 diabetes. Elevated insulin triggers the release of additional testosterone, which worsens acne, facial hair, and irregular periods. Sleep deprivation increases cortisol as well, which causes irritability, aggression, and anger. Stress and anxiety are the result of cortisol.

Studies show that people who are sleep-deprived tend to crave foods that are high in sugar and fats. This is partly a physiological response to insulin resistance but is also due to the effect of sleep deprivation on ghrelin and leptin. *Ghrelin* is also known as the hunger hormone—it tells us when we need to eat again. Levels of ghrelin are elevated even after just one night of too-little sleep, meaning our appetites skyrocket when we're overtired.[2] *Leptin* is a hormone that is created in the fat cells. Its job is to help the body stay at a healthy weight. Typically, where there is more fat, there is also more leptin to send the body signals that it is full. However, when a body is sleep-deprived, leptin levels actually drop, leaving you feeling like you're starving, even if you've eaten adequately all day!

Sleep also supports the development of muscle mass and helps repair cells. This is important not only if we want to see results from all our hard work in the gym but also because the heart, being a muscle, is affected by sleep deprivation as well. And your body needs sleep for a healthy immune system. Sleep deficiency over the long run can lead to an immune system that is weak and could eventually lead to autoimmune disease.

Sleep deprivation is associated with elevated levels of *C-reactive protein*, or CRP—a substance produced by the liver that increases when there is inflammation in the body, effectively serving as a signal that there is something wrong in the body. Lack of sleep can elevate CRP as much as can a diet containing processed foods and sugar. CRP is a significant risk factor for heart disease and is related to the development of PCOS. Metformin therapy reduces CRP level and the related high glucose; however, *lifestyle change is the first line of treatment for elevated CRP levels and PCOS.*[3]

The physical effects of sleep deprivation aren't just internal; they can affect your safety in completing your job and everyday tasks as well. Sleep deprivation can also lead to *microsleeps* throughout the day—tiny, almost unnoticeable mininaps during which you zone out. Have you ever driven somewhere and yet don't really remember getting there? Or perhaps you listened to a lecture in class and but somehow missed a big part of it? You could have been experiencing a microsleep.

Lack of sleep also affects psychological health. People with chronic sleep deprivation are more likely to suffer from depression and anxiety. They may also suffer from mood swings and problems with attention. Depression and anxiety can result from sleep deprivation due to desensitized serotonin receptors (serotonin contributes to a sense of well-being and happiness). What that means is that even if there is serotonin in the system, it can't be used.

One study found that once serotonin receptors were desensitized, the system didn't go back to normal for at least a week. This is one reason why you can't deprive yourself of sleep all week and then hope to make up for it on weekends.

Sleep is broken up into three basic parts: light sleep, deep sleep, and REM sleep.

REM sleep—This sleep phase is named for the characteristic rapid eye movements that occur during this stage and is the stage of sleep that is most often associated with dreams. We spend about 25 percent of our sleeping in REM sleep. The brain waves produced when we are in REM are similar to the brain waves produced when we are awake. Lack of REM sleep leads to a subsequent inability to complete complex tasks in waking. Memories are also organized during this stage of sleep, so memory can be affected if REM is interrupted. Sufficient REM sleep allows you to feel energized the next morning.

Light sleep—This is when the body drifts easily in and out of sleep, and it comprises about half of an adult's sleep time.

Deep sleep—It is during this phase that we are most unaware of our surroundings. Phases of deep sleep occur more in the first half of the night and are when the body releases growth hormones for muscle building and repair; it is believed to be the most restorative sleep.

Understanding the different phases of sleep and their purposes and impacts on us can help us better understand our body's function, which, in turn, can help us best figure out what we need to do to create and support healthier sleep patterns. I recommend keeping a sleep journal: On a notepad by your bed, record the time you went to bed and the time you wake up. Or consider purchasing a wearable activity tracker that monitors your sleep and heart rate; this gives you more detailed information about your total time asleep and the duration of each sleep cycle.

While we may understand and accept that sufficient uninterrupted sleep is critical to our wellness, we still may not be very good yet at *getting* sufficient, uninterrupted sleep. But there are a few tweaks we can make to personal habits that can make it easier to fall asleep quickly, deeply, and when we need to. Sleep hygiene is most commonly disrupted by the following:

In the hours just prior to bed using a device like a phone or tablet—
Sleeping with your device close by can actually reinforce anxiety

and fear that you'll miss an important e-mail at 2 AM. Sleeping with your device near your bed also increases the likelihood that you will check your phone when you wake up in the middle of the night, which disrupts sleep cycles. In addition, the blue light is emitted from these devices also stimulates the release of cortisol, which in turn further disrupts sleep patterns. The solution? The National Sleep Foundation recommends turning off all devices one hour before bedtime. This is because the blue light blocks the release of melatonin, which is critical to helping you fall asleep.[4]

Drinking midafternoon coffee or "energy" drinks—The effectiveness of caffeine lasts about four to six hours, so a morning cup or two is unlikely to have an effect on sleep. Not so for caffeinated beverages later in the day. Instead, try getting some fresh air or having a stretch; it might be a better way to get through any midafternoon slump without compromising your ability to fall asleep that night.[5]

Erratic sleep schedule—Try to fall asleep and wake up at the same time each day; reinforcing this pattern helps the body fall more naturally and easily into sustained sleep at a predictable time.

SLEEP SOLUTIONS

Getting good sleep is a learned skill to be developed. Unfortunately, we tend to develop coping strategies to avoid the discipline of an effective sleep routine.

Sleep medications—Should you take them? Numerous medications and supplements are available to help you fall asleep and stay asleep. That said, chronic lack of sleep is often an indicator that your lifestyle needs adjustment.

Naps—Are they helpful? While the research behind the benefits of taking a nap are extensive and generally positive, the need for a daily nap might signal the need to give more attention to the evening sleep routine. That said, if you enjoy a midafternoon nap, go ahead; just keep it brief, forty-five minutes or less, and you should get a fantastic energy boost without disrupting sleep later.

So, how do we turn this around and learn good sleep hygiene?

Think happy thoughts . . . the right way—Make those happy thoughts work for you. This suggestion is handy, because it's something you can do with no equipment or prep work. Thoughts combined with emotion make for powerful behavior change. Think of a time that filled your heart with happiness. Maybe it's the day you met your spouse. Or that time you went to a Red Sox game with your dad. Make sure to choose a memory that doesn't trigger any negative feelings. Next, go over it detail by detail, from start to finish, like watching it on a video. The more specific you are in working through this memory, the more powerful it will be, so resist the urge to gloss over any parts of the story. The more you practice this relaxation technique, the less time it will take for your brain to switch gears and drift off to sleep.

Plan ahead for morning success—One of the hardest things about falling asleep is our tendency to think about all the things we need to do the next day. Allay some of these anxieties by doing what you can to get a jump on tomorrow's list, thereby setting yourself up for success the night before. For example, if getting to the gym is on your list the following day, lay out your exercise clothes that night. If just getting out the door is difficult for you every morning, try to prep for breakfast the night before to save you some time and stress. Putting into place simple, effective solutions to lessen the next day's anxieties can make it easier to relax into sleep.

Write it down—But what about the million things buzzing through your head that you know you have to do? What you can't accomplish the night before, write down on a list that you keep by your bedside table. Just knowing that you have noted it is often enough to allow your brain to relax so that you can sleep.

Exercise—Since anxiety is one of the main causes of sleeplessness, the calming effects of exercise can be enormously helpful to people who struggle with sleep. Any exercise will do, from yoga to taking the dog for a brisk walk.

Don't overthink it—Keep a relaxed mind-set about sleep. You don't want to make your prebedtime routine so complex that it is impossible to accomplish consistently. Don't think in terms of "making" yourself go to sleep. Instead, "allow" yourself to sleep.

Eat a snack (yes, even after 8 PM)—You may have heard some advice on the Internet to stop eating at a certain time of night, but let's face it: your appetite doesn't have a watch. Fighting with your appetite just before bed is a recipe for sleeplessness. Your metabolism does slow down while you sleep, but not so drastically that having a small, healthy snack before bed should cause concern. If you're hungry, have a light snack, and then go to bed without beating yourself up.

Create a routine, and be consistent—You might have heard that it takes twenty-one days to form a habit. This may be true, but what you may not know is that first you have to find the right habit to form! It's okay to guess and check when you're trying a new sleep routine. Try something for a few days before going to the next approach. It may take a while to find what works for you—longer than twenty-one days. Just don't give up on the idea of better sleep.

Cuddle up—Cuddling with your favorite person releases oxytocin, the hormone responsible for the loving connections you feel with family and close friends. Cuddling also lowers cortisol, which makes it a benefit to your overall health.

Avoid overindulging in alcohol—While there is nothing wrong with having a drink, alcohol consumption could be affecting your sleep more than you think! Many people mistakenly think that alcohol will *help* them sleep, but this is problematic thinking for a few reasons. First, alcohol can disrupt normal sleep cycles, meaning you won't wake up refreshed. Second, too much alcohol can cause the liver to kick into overdrive in order to clear it out; the liver works the hardest around 2 AM, and if it has to work too hard, then it will likely wake you up. Third, add to that the dose of anxiety you're bound to get from being awakened at 2 AM without understanding why, and you're probably not getting back to sleep anytime soon. So, avoid alcohol within three hours of bedtime.

Practice gratitude—Whether you are a glass-half-full or glass-half-empty sort of person, you will definitely feel better if you take some time in your day to cultivate gratitude. Even if things are tough right now, being grateful for the learning experiences is both powerful and calming. If your mind wanders to either solving the problem or getting grumpy about it, let go of that thought and gently bring your focus back to gratitude.

JOURNAL QUESTIONS

1. What are three things you can do to make your bedroom a better environment for sleep?
2. What are your sleep habits? How do they vary from one night to the next? Are weekends different?
3. How will your health improve with better sleep?
4. What is your preferred way to track your sleep?
5. What prebedtime strategies can you implement? (Focus on the last hour before sleep.)

5

❖ ❖

Anxiety

It's Not All in Your Head

A nxiety is a normal emotion that can serve a useful purpose. Unfortunately, it can sometimes get out of control and become problematic.
A variety of effective treatment options address anxiety disorders—the
most common mental health issue in the United States[1]—including lifestyle changes, nutritional adjustments, therapy, and medication. If you
struggle with anxiety, I want you to know that you aren't going crazy and
you're not alone.

The American Psychological Association defines *anxiety* as "an emotion characterized by feelings of tension, worried thoughts, and physical
changes, like increased blood pressure. People with anxiety disorders usually have recurring intrusive thoughts or concerns. They may avoid certain
situations out of worry. They may also have physical symptoms such as
sweating, trembling, dizziness, or a rapid heartbeat."[2]

Women with PCOS are at increased risk for anxiety. This is likely a
result of the double-whammy that the syndrome hits us with: On one
hand, anxiety can be caused by the symptoms and effects of PCOS, such
as thinning hair, excessive facial and body hair, cystic acne, weight gain,
difficulty losing weight, and infertility. On the other hand, anxiety can be
caused by nutritional deficiencies resulting from excessively long menstrual cycles, high levels of glucose, and medications like metformin and
birth control pills. The degree to which you suffer from anxiety can vary;
however, the most important thing to know is that anxiety is a normal
reaction to a cocktail of stressors including cortisol imbalance, overthinking, and stale energy. Generalized anxiety is often caused by a disconnect

between where you are and where you want to be in your work, life, and relationships. Some people are just more prone to anxiety.

This chapter explains these issues and offers targeted solutions so that you can start to feel better. If you do have anxiety along with PCOS, I recommend that you start your journey to wellness here and get your anxiety to a manageable level. Doing so will free up emotional energy so that you can tackle other lifestyle changes that might take you outside of your comfort zone.

There is a growing trend of body-positive activism, which is wonderful; however, some women feel as though they've failed if they don't love everything about facial hair and acne. While I do believe that it's important to love yourself and your body, if anxiety is caused by your feelings about the symptoms of PCOS, like some of the more difficult physical presentations, then it is helpful to take action and address them without feeling guilty about it. It is absolutely possible to love yourself fully and also want better health.

If you are on a medication that you feel might be contributing to your anxiety, I strongly recommend that you talk with your health-care provider before making any changes. Some medications have uncomfortable and even dangerous side effects when they are stopped suddenly. Also, because some supplements can have adverse reactions to medications, be sure to discuss supplements with your doctor as well. If your anxiety results from your feelings about managing the difficult symptoms of PCOS, the best way to start feeling better is to do something about it. Whether you are partnering with your doctor or you're going this alone, the strategies in this book will help you establish yourself as the key player when it comes to the long-term management of your PCOS.

The National Institute of Mental Health reports that anxiety is the most common mental illness in the population, with 18 percent of adults experiencing it at some point in their lives. The rate is even higher among women with PCOS. Anxiety can manifest in physical symptoms or in mental symptoms, such as irritability or an inability to concentrate. Many people who have anxiety aren't entirely aware that they have it. To some people, life just feels harder, but since anxiety disorders can start at a very young age, it's hard to know what's "normal" and what is disordered anxiety.

In talking about mental health and PCOS, anxiety and depression are very often lumped together. While anxiety and depression do sometimes occur together, they are experienced very differently and deserve to be considered separately. (See chapter 6 for an extended discussion of depression.)

Stress and *anxiety* are terms that are also used interchangeably. While some of the physical effects are similar, it's important to be able to identify the difference to manage them properly. Anxiety is persistent worry or dread about something that may not actually be a threat. Stress is a reaction to an actual situation. Generally, when the stressor is removed, the stress passes. It only becomes a problem when the stress is long term. (More on stress in chapter 8.)

IN YOUR MIND

Anxiety can feel like a whirlwind of what-ifs. You may get stuck worrying and have difficulty progressing to active problem-solving. Being told to calm down is, at best, ineffective and can actually make anxiety worse by attaching shame to the experience.

IN YOUR BODY

Physically, anxiety can be experienced as stomachaches, headaches, digestive problems, or tightness in the chest that feels similar to a heart attack. You might feel restless, or, at the other end of the spectrum, you might feel unable to move. Identifying your body's response to anxiety can help you understand what's happening to you when it occurs. If you don't know whether you are having a panic attack or a heart attack, call 911; the symptoms are so similar that it may take a medical diagnosis to be sure.

WHAT OTHERS SEE

Sadly, most people don't notice that you're feeling anxious. If anything, they might think that you're aloof or overly serious. Studies have shown that people with social anxiety overestimate the potential for negative reactions from those with whom they are interacting.

WHAT'S ACTUALLY HAPPENING

I find it's helpful to think of anxiety as an emotion, not a diagnosis. Anxiety is a valid feeling and can have useful applications. It is an indicator to others that we are genuine and approachable. It also helps us identify trouble so that we stay safe. The problem is when the anxiety becomes intrusive. If your anxiety begins to feel overwhelming, you should not hesitate to get help.

While anxiety can happen to anyone, a study by Columbia University School of Nursing found that, for women with PCOS, lack of periods caused more emotional distress than any other symptom.[3] While it's certainly understandable that the outward signs of PCOS can create anxiety, another theory is that there is a biological cause.

Medications like birth control pills and metformin can reduce B vitamins in the body. B-vitamin deficiency can cause anxiety, as B vitamins are essential to converting the food-based nutrient tryptophan into serotonin (the brain's feel-good chemical).

While many women with PCOS don't regularly have a period, others will have periods that last for months. In this case, it is important to look at iron levels, as iron deficiency has been associated with anxiety disorders as well.

TREATMENT OPTIONS

Anxiety is very treatable, and there is a lot that a physician or mental-health worker can do to help you resolve your anxiety. Blood tests can be done to check for most nutritional deficiencies. Although this book is primarily about lifestyle strategies, there are a number of medications that are incredibly effective in easing anxiety. Medications are sometimes necessary, and there is nothing unhealthy about taking them when you need them. I encourage you to talk with your doctor about your options. In focusing on lifestyle strategies, I in no way mean to diminish the effectiveness of professional help. It is imperative that you get the help that you need. You don't need to wait until you are suffering terribly or in a crisis situation. Treating anxiety early can reduce the negative impact it has over your life.

Cognitive behavioral therapy—or CBT—is arguably the most effective therapeutic approach to treating anxiety. It tends to be a short-term, structured therapeutic approach that addresses the way a person perceives and reacts to a situation and then helps them develop new thinking patterns and behaviors aligned with that new perception. Often just a few sessions of CBT can ease suffering.

I firmly believe that the most powerful results to treating anxiety come from a multidisciplinary approach—meaning, pulling strategies, tools, and knowledge from all available resources and using them in a way that is right for you. Just like the various medications that treat PCOS, these lifestyle strategies can also be helpful when used in conjunction with professional intervention. Conversely, ignoring these strategies and relying solely on medication is likely to result in reduced effectiveness and a longer time spent in treatment.[4] Medication is generally a last resort and should always be used in conjunction with therapy and lifestyle changes; lifestyle strategies like healthy eating habits, consistent exercise, staying hydrated, and getting adequate sleep can also improve most types of anxiety.[5]

Anxiety is an umbrella term for a wide range of issues. It's important to understand what type of anxiety you have in order to address it properly. Anxiety affects more than 18 percent of the adult population in the United States.[6] If your anxiety is bothersome but you're not ready for professional help, I encourage you to build some of these strategies into your daily life:

Avoid alcohol—Alcohol depletes B vitamins, which in turn can reduce blood-sugar control and block the production of serotonin. Because alcohol is processed in the liver, it impairs the production of glucose, which can then lead to low blood sugar, even twelve hours after drinking.[7] Either avoid alcohol altogether or limit yourself to one serving of alcohol per day to avoid negative effects.

Watch your blood sugar—Levels that are too high or too low can trigger feelings of anxiety. You can manage this by eating regular meals that include complex carbohydrates and protein.

Eat foods that contain tryptophan—Turkey, sunflower seeds, and egg whites are among the foods that contain this serotonin-creating amino acid.

SEROTONIN

Serotonin is a neurotransmitter that is produced in the brain and intestines. It is also known as the "feel-good chemical" because of the part it plays in elevating moods. From a lifestyle-strategies standpoint, our goal is to manage serotonin levels in two ways: foods that boost serotonin are helpful, but it is equally important to do what you can to prevent serotonin from being depleted in the first place. That said, if you find that your medications are depleting serotonin, talk to your doctor before discontinuing them.

TRYPTOPHAN

Tryptophan is an amino acid found in food that is necessary in the production of serotonin. Generally, a balanced and varied diet provides enough tryptophan to maintain healthy levels of serotonin in the body, but when there are other factors that deplete the serotonin in the body, it's helpful to be aware of foods high in tryptophan to incorporate into your diet, including:

eggs, with yolks
cheese
soy products, like tofu, tempeh, soy milk, and meat replacements
salmon
nuts and seeds
turkey
inositol, though not a food, is one supplement that has been found to
    boost serotonin and has benefits for regulating blood sugar and lower-
    ing testosterone

MAGNESIUM

Magnesium deficiency is very common in women with PCOS due to the effect of birth control pills, eating simple sugars, and high levels of glucose in the blood. All of these things deplete the body of magnesium, which can then trigger anxiety and worsen inflammation within the body.[8] Sources of magnesium in food are generally tolerated better than magnesium supplements, which can cause diarrhea.[9] Some food sources include:

spinach
chard
dark chocolate
pumpkin seeds
almonds
yogurt
black beans

EXERCISE AND ANXIETY

Consistent daily exercise is the best bet when it comes to beating anxiety. One study found that yoga is more effective than walking when it comes to decreasing anxiety. While light cardio has numerous other physiological benefits, it's important to decide what exercise is best for you. If your anxiety is the most uncomfortable part of your life right now and yoga helps, then definitely do yoga. You can always change or add cardio to the mix later on.

The Role of Exercise in Managing Anxiety

Research indicates that, when it comes to reducing general anxiety, exercise can be as effective as medication for most people.[10] The interesting thing is that it doesn't take an incredible amount of time to exercise every day. While you may end up wanting to work out longer for other reasons, just ten minutes of exercise can have a positive psychophysiological effect. One study of people suffering headache compared the effects of a short workout to the effects of taking an aspirin, finding that both alleviated pain for up to several hours. Consistent exercise has even shown to have a preventative effect against anxiety. This is great news for people who have struggled with some form of chronic anxiety. Often, women with anxiety are told to *quit worrying so much*, but it's not all in your head, and you generally can't just jolly your way through it. You don't have to suffer with it though. Lifestyle changes like exercise are powerful healers—especially for women who have PCOS.

CORTISOL, OVERTHINKING, AND ANXIETY

Cortisol levels that are out of balance can trigger feelings of anxiety. It has been suggested that you can, with the help of your doctor, replace the cortisol and feel better, but there are several problems with this medical intervention. First, the symptoms of too-high cortisol and too-low cortisol are very similar and difficult to differentiate. Chronic stress leads to elevated cortisol levels but will eventually lead to what is referred to as *adrenal fatigue*. Basically, your body is exhausted from trying to keep pumping out cortisol, and as a result your cortisol level drops dramatically.

The other problem with cortisol replacement is that it is simply a Band-Aid for a larger underlying problem that must be solved first in order for you to be healthy. Diet and exercise are a vital part of this solution, as is learning to deal constructively with chronically stressful situations. While perfection is impossible, simple behavioral shifts in these areas can tip the scales and bring your cortisol level to somewhere within the normal range.

But it's not all cortisol's fault. Sometimes an anxiety-provoking situation is created by overthinking—a habit that comes in the form of racing thoughts. You have an anxious thought, and you respond to it with a cascade of worries that build on one another. These thoughts haven't been reality checked. It's like a stream of consciousness fueled by worry. Mindfulness, staying present, and being aware of your thoughts as they flow through you are beneficial. This may sound like a lot of whimsy, but there is evidence to back it up. A recent study found that mindfulness-based techniques had a similar, if not better, effect on anxiety when compared to the effects of cognitive behavioral therapy.[11]

SO OVERWHELMED YOU DON'T KNOW WHERE TO BEGIN?

The key to eliminating anxiety is two-fold: First, diet, exercise, and lifestyle change to address nutritional deficiencies is powerful and can dramatically reduce the chemical cause of anxiety. Second, mindfulness techniques are useful to breaking the cycle of overthinking. Learn to be present. Essentially, you want to get more comfortable sitting with the anxiety for a moment. Does that mean that you have to strike a meditation pose every time you feel stressed? Definitely not! Like a hypnotist snapping someone out of a trance, I want to you learn to snap yourself out of your racing thoughts. Acknowledging them essentially whisks the rug out from under them. This takes practice, but you'll likely get plenty of opportunity, as racing thoughts tend to have a predictable story line.

RECHANNELING ANXIETY

Many people have established scripts for some of their most common insecurities. Women with PCOS often have a script of what other people might think or say about cystic acne or excessive facial hair.

You may be tempted to think that anxiety is a weakness, but actually, with the right perspective, you can come to see that it's a superpower: Anxiety is nothing more than stale energy. Energy is meant to move and flow. When there are blocks in life, that energy can't flow. It gets stuck, and then we experience it as frustration, which quickly goes stale. The result is anxiety. But the very existence of anxiety at all is an indication of your stores of energy and power.

When you catch yourself playing out an anxious script, you can choose to stop it. First, acknowledge that you are working off a script. Play detective: What evidence do you have that what you are worrying about will even happen? Slow your thoughts down a bit. Sitting with the anxiety gives you more time to fact-check it.

Now exercise. Daily exercise has a powerful effect on anxiety. It distracts you from your script and then burns off excess blood sugar, which then allows for better-regulated cortisol levels.[12] And exercise feels empowering. It improves creativity and helps you identify what fulfills you. Anxiety is energy, so try to choose something that will release that energy. Challenge yourself with your exercise, but stay within your personal health limits—don't underestimate the power of an evening walk!

For women with PCOS, anxiety requires a combination of mind-set shift, to slow runaway thinking, and consistent exercise, to burn off the energy that is created.

BENEFITS OF ANXIETY?

Anxiety in its intended form is a normal and helpful reaction to an unusual situation. At healthy levels, anxiety can provide a boost of clarity. For example, you are more likely to get the whole picture of a situation by looking at all of the pros and cons rather than by focusing solely only on the positives. This can be incredibly helpful when you're deciding whether to buy a new house or whether to take that new job in another city. Healthy levels of anxiety can also boost creativity. This is applicable to problem solving as well as artistic endeavors, and with more problem-solving skills come more options in figuring out how to deal with what life throws your way. Anxiety can also boost performance when you learn to control it and not let it make you choke. Unfortunately, most of us will tolerate unacceptable levels of anxiety for ages before we take action to control it or even define it.

WHY IT'S NOT OKAY TO TOUGH IT OUT

Just because you can tolerate something doesn't mean you should. The consequences to unchecked anxiety have a wide and scary reach. As a rule, human beings are efficient problem solvers. Unfortunately, in our rush to feel better, we may not choose the healthiest coping strategy. Things like food, sex, and drugs are all ways to cope with anxiety, sure, but they only mask the symptoms and can come with their own perils: food addiction, drug addiction, alcoholism, and obsessive compulsive disorder are all attempts to resolve anxiety. These behaviors become a diagnosis when they become the lone tool in the bag of coping strategies. The bad news is that if healthy strategies aren't introduced, the anxiety will likely get worse. This happens because of the process that creates the anxiety: If you experience an anxiety and the situation that caused it has either ended (e.g., airplane ride is over or the public speech has concluded) or been masked (with alcohol, binge eating, or drugs) before it's been healthily acknowledged and coped with, then you have merely taught yourself to white-knuckle it through anxiety instead of productively managing it. The next time an anxious episode comes around, you're trained to tolerate that anxiety as a part of the natural course of things instead of knowing how to decrease or even stop it altogether. Basically, you've taught yourself to experience anxiety for longer periods of time.

There is a "sweet spot" for anxiety when it comes to all of the positive benefits mentioned earlier. Going beyond that level of anxiety results in a drastic loss of usefulness and can lead to health problems. Excessive anxiety can limit your lifestyle. Social anxiety is a common type of anxiety for women with PCOS. While it could be related to suffering from the symptoms of the disorder, it could also be due to a B-vitamin and zinc deficiency. And anxiety can reinforce itself as a coping strategy. The more frequently overanxious episodes occur without being productively addressed, the more anxiety becomes your norm whenever the going gets tough.

Then, over time, your immune system is weakened; perhaps this means you catch every cold or flu that comes through your office. Your fight-or-flight response is compromised; you can't stay in a heightened state of emergency readiness without some kind of burnout. Often this results in adrenal fatigue.

If you're wired for anxiety, you have to learn to manage it right along with your PCOS. Fortunately, what's good for one is almost always good for the other, so suffering from anxiety is really just another reason to adopt a healthy lifestyle.

Coping strategies are methods that are developed to reduce or avoid the discomfort from anxiety. There are several factors that determine whether a person will choose an active, problem-solving approach or an avoidant approach. Basically, this book is about identifying active coping strategies for your PCOS. The attempt is to problem solve without causing additional emotional pain. Unfortunately, many avoidance strategies don't solve the problem, which is likely to make the anxiety worse as time passes. Since consistent exercise and a healthy diet improve creative problem solving, developing a healthy lifestyle can create a positive cycle for lasting health.

NEGATIVE AVOIDANCE STRATEGIES FOR ANXIETY

Many people suffering from anxiety will form negative coping skills that may seem like they help in the short run but instead often actually become problems of their own. Here are some common, yet unhelpful, ways people try to soothe their anxiety.

Food—Binge eating is a common coping strategy for anxiety and is especially troublesome for women with PCOS because food choices are an important part of managing insulin resistance. That said, being a binge eater is not an identity, and I do not believe that it should be a diagnosis. It is a coping strategy.[13] In fact, all of these behaviors are simply tools in the toolbox of coping strategies. I'll explain binge eating at length in the next section, but for now, suffice it to say that if you binge eat, you're not alone.

Alcohol—Drinking is a culturally accepted method of blocking social anxiety, which is a very common type of anxiety for women with PCOS. While one glass of dry (low-sugar) wine can be part of a healthy lifestyle, heavy drinking should be avoided, as it can actually trigger anxiety and even panic attacks. Alcohol strips the body of B vitamins.

Cigarettes—Smoking depletes your body of vitamins B_5 and B_{12}. B_5 is necessary for heart health and the formation of red blood cells that carry oxygen throughout the body; this is important if you are at risk for anemia. Vitamin B_{12} has many uses, including converting carbohydrates into glucose (blood sugar) for energy. Women who smoke should put quitting smoking at the top of their get-healthy to-do list.

Drugs—Addiction is chronic, progressive, and often fatal. If you're on drugs, you must address that first before thinking about your PCOS. That said, healthy lifestyle strategies can be helpful when used along with a drug-treatment program.

Anxious Eating: What You Need to Know

There are a lot of reasons why people overeat. The most common is eating to control anxiety.

The first thing you need to know is that, while overeating may not be ideal, it's normal! From a biological standpoint, it's logical: Different foods will trigger chemical responses in our bodies that relieve pain, depression, and anxiety. You can think of overeating as self-medicating. The trouble starts when overeating becomes the go-to strategy for managing anxiety.

Anxiety calls for more attention when it starts to limit your activities and relationships. It also deserves to be addressed when it continues despite resulting in negative health consequences, such as overweight, diabetes, or allergic responses. This is a compounded problem for women with PCOS. Not only does sugar go straight to the reward part of the brain much like drugs do (this is true for everyone), but for women with PCOS sugar also leads to dangerous spikes in blood sugar that cause brain fog, weakness, inflammation, and hormone imbalances. This all then leads to more anxiety, creating a vicious cycle: overeating—blood-sugar spike—stressful and negative health effects—overeating to self-soothe. When you find yourself munching in an anxious state, acknowledge what you're doing. No judgment, no self-hate. Just notice. You might even say to yourself, *I notice that I'm feeling anxious and am overeating as a result.*

Many people who use food as a way to cope with anxiety make the mistake of trying to control their eating habits instead of managing their anxiety. The more effective approach is to remove the cause of the anxiety. Relief might come from a simple shift in perspective or a conversation that you've been putting off. It could require professional help with a skilled counselor to release some feelings that have been locked into your experience for a long time. Either way, the return on that investment is nothing short of miraculous for many people. If the anxiety is resolved, the need for food to "treat" the anxiety is no longer relevant. The physical and emotional benefits of this type of healing are profound and well worth the effort.

Binge eating might be a problem if you are

eating more than would be considered normal
feeling remorse after eating
binge eating at least once a week for at least three months

What Is the Cycle of Binge Eating?

Binge eating typically follows a familiar progression:

Before the binge—Insulin resistance can cause significant cravings, making it quite common among women with PCOS. There could also be a history of family fights or feelings of powerlessness surrounding food. This scenario places food in a highly emotional part of the brain rather than letting us properly contextualize it: as a nutritional or cultural key. Eating then becomes a go-to coping strategy when emotional pressure builds. Keep in mind that the typical food craving lasts about fifteen minutes. To break the habit, try to acknowledge the craving and choose to do something else for fifteen minutes. Journaling during these times is incredibly powerful and can provide valuable insight. Even if you end up binge eating, you learn a lot in those fifteen minutes. Practiced over time, you will have a deeper understanding of yourself and strong emotional resiliency, which can help alleviate the need to binge eat.

During the binge—There is pressure to eat with the intent to calm negative feelings. You might feel sick to your stomach or shaky and anxious from elevated sugar in your bloodstream.

After the binge—Typically, feelings of guilt and regret follow a binge. Negative self-talk erodes self-esteem and wears down the belief that change from within is possible.

Binge eating can be hard to treat with the typical addictions model because it's impossible to abstain from food as it would be with alcohol or drugs. You can, however, choose to limit sugar and simple carbohydrates with no risk to nutrition. I recommend that you don't go after the binge eating because it is just the byproduct of anxiety. Always look for the source of the anxiety and start there. Daily exercise can reduce anxiety and depression and increase confidence and self-esteem. Staying hydrated will also help. Learning to set boundaries with anything or anyone who has a negative impact on your life is imperative. Always ask for help when you need it. I do recommend that you avoid online binge-eating support groups. These are rarely well moderated and generally contain posts of repeated binge-eating behavior that may be triggering. Most women I have worked with find that their energy and resolve to stay on target with their goals disintegrates in these groups. Instead, talk to an understanding friend or, even better, a counselor.

PUTTING THE PIECES TOGETHER
TO MANAGE ANXIETY

Start with what's doable: Identify your triggers, and map out possible solutions. If changing your diet seems like too much to try, start with a daily ten-minute walk. Make a list of questions about your vitamins and where you think there might be deficiencies so you can talk to your doctor about supplements.

Feeling anxious? Here are some strategies to use right now:

Mindfulness meditation apps—Use them daily as part of your wellness routine and any time you notice your anxiety increasing.

Deep breathing—In through the nose, out through the mouth.

Noticing the little things—The feeling of your toes pressing into the floor. Or look for ten things that are in your favorite color.

Shaking it out—Move your arms and legs, and gently twist at your waist while making a yawning motion with your jaw to loosen muscles you may not have been aware you were clenching.

Water—Have a glass.

Outside time—Go outside for five minutes, especially if it's sunny outside, as the sun can help with vitamin D production.

Counting sounds—If you're in a safe place to do so, close your eyes and count the number of sounds you hear. Do you hear the air conditioner, the hum of the refrigerator, the birds outside? Make sure you're breathing deeply as you do this.

Prayer—If you're spiritual, this can be an effective strategy, as it lifts the burden of worrying.

JOURNAL QUESTIONS

1. What are all of the emotions you are feeling right now? It's important to simply list them, maybe even describe them, but don't judge them.
2. What are all of the things you have accomplished today? No success is too small. It is all relevant. If you journal in the morning, list your accomplishments from the day before.
3. What activity helps you manage your anxiety? How can you do that more often?
4. What situations trigger your anxiety? Describe them. Do you notice any trends? How can you disrupt the anxiety either before, during, or after?

6

❖ ❖

Depression

You Can *Feel Better*

L ike anxiety, *depression* is a term that gets tossed around freely in our language and culture. When most people say they are depressed, they often mean that they are feeling sad, lethargic, or bummed out. We use the word *depression* fairly loosely to describe anything from a mild case of the blues to a sometimes-crippling mental-health issue, which is why so many well-intentioned people simply don't know how to help when we say we are depressed.

From a clinical standpoint, there are several different types of depression. Those most often linked to PCOS are major depressive disorder (MDD) and persistent depressive disorder (PDD). MDD, the more severe of the two, is the most common reason for disability claims in the United States, affecting about 5 percent of the US population, and is more common among women than men.[1] PDD is a somewhat milder form of depression; however, for a diagnosis to be made, it must be present for more than two years. While this condition only affects 1.5 percent of the population, its effects can be devastating.[2]

Most people feel sad or "depressed" at one time or another, and typically this is due to an external, experiential occurrence, such as a death in the family or the loss of a job. This is a normal reaction to real life. Typically, this type of sadness has a specific cause, and the feelings resolve over time.

However, some people feel the same feelings more frequently and without a specific cause. Women often express feelings of sadness, irritability, and more; yet they don't know why. This type of depressive suffering is similar to anxiety, because it is incredibly confusing for the sufferer and her loved ones to understand and cope when a normal emotion that should ebb and flow with the circumstances becomes the default emotion. With true depression, there's often not a particular event that causes the feeling to occur; it just happens. The line between "feeling down" and clinical depression is drawn when the feeling begins to affect your health, safety, and quality of life.

Nearly half of people diagnosed with depression are also diagnosed with anxiety disorder, so the diagnoses can overlap.[3] This is not only at the point where it is severe enough to be a diagnosable mental illness but also before it is severe enough to become a diagnosis. It is important to understand the differences between anxiety and depression, however, as they have different impacts on life.

Symptoms of major depressive disorder include feeling sad or empty. MDD sufferers often ask, *What's the point?* and feel guilty, helpless, or as though they are not good enough. They might lose interest in activities that they once found enjoyable. Physical symptoms of MDD are similar to anxiety: headaches, stomach upset, or unexplained and untreatable aches and pains. Fatigue is a very common symptom. Difficulty concentrating and making decisions can also occur. Sleep patterns are disrupted, and a person with MDD can have insomnia or will sleep too much. Changes in eating patterns are a red flag. At its extreme, people with MDD may contemplate or even attempt suicide. If you are thinking of harming yourself or committing suicide, get help now! Go to the emergency room, contact your mental-health provider, and call the Suicide Prevention Lifeline immediately.[4]

Persistent depressive disorder usually continues for at least two years. While not as intense or deep as MDD, PDD involves some of the same symptoms, which include low energy, irritability, poor appetite or overeating, insomnia, and a loss of pleasure over things once enjoyed. Because PDD is long term, the far-reaching effects on health, relationships, and motivation can cause a huge impact.

Just like anxiety, one of the most common therapies for any type of depression is cognitive behavioral therapy. Treatment for depression typically takes a bit longer than for anxiety, but treatment duration can vary from person to person. There are other therapeutic approaches that might be helpful, including medications prescribed by a psychiatrist. It's important to work with a therapist you can connect with and like and who is open and experienced in the therapeutic approach you're most comfortable with.

The suggestions in this book are not intended to take the place of medical or psychological advice; they are meant to help you achieve the lifestyle changes that are a part of any recommended therapy or treatment. That said, there is a distinct benefit to pursuing a healthy lifestyle while you are *also* pursuing medicinal or psychological intervention. Doing so will elevate the therapeutic effectiveness. Be sure to mention to your mental-health provider that you are working toward better health overall, and discuss supplements or concerns about medication.

THE LINK BETWEEN PCOS AND DEPRESSION

Much as they are more likely than the general population to suffer from anxiety, women with PCOS are at a greater risk of depression.[5] The onset of depression can be a response to a particular situation, but there could also be a biochemical factor to it that is exciting in that effective treatments are possible.

Many studies have confirmed a link between insulin resistance and depression.[6] Unfortunately, many women manage to endure PCOS symptoms but are so troubled by depression that they seek psychological intervention. If you have depression and PCOS, talk to your provider about medications to control insulin resistance.

There is also a link between elevated cortisol levels and depression and another link between elevated cortisol and insulin resistance. Insulin resistance and overweight are also linked. Fortunately, it is possible to disrupt this connection with the right combination of lifestyle changes and medication for insulin resistance.

THE ROLE OF CORTISOL

Cortisol gets a bad rap as the stress hormone, but it actually serves a vital function, creating more glucose in the bloodstream when we come under stress—just in case we need it for the fight-or-flight response.

For women who live chronically stressed lives, however, cortisol is a problem, in that it creates more glucose than the body needs—because, let's face it, the kind of stress we typically endure is more emotional than physical. Being stressed about work-life balance is a far cry from running away from a pack of wild animals. This overload of unused glucose leads to inflammation and exacerbates other problems like insulin resistance, excess facial hair, and acne. Women with PCOS are particularly at risk for the ill effects of chronic stress and the resulting excess cortisol because, with insulin resistance, glucose is trapped in the bloodstream even longer than in women without insulin resistance.

Ideal treatment for PCOS will address elevated cortisol levels in addition to insulin resistance and other symptoms of PCOS from several different approaches. Medicines like metformin and spironolactone can improve insulin resistance and decrease the related acne and hirsutism. The best treatment for PCOS, however, is to support medical interventions with lifestyle changes.

LIFESTYLE CHANGES FOR DEPRESSION RELIEF

To understand depression from a lifestyle perspective, it's important to know that depression is a normal response to an abnormal situation. Having PCOS is tough, especially in the beginning. It's absolutely true that depression is anger turned inward and anger is sad's bodyguard, and you're probably sad or angry about the effects of PCOS, so your depression is a logical progression.

Logical, but not effective.

Fortunately, depression caused by anger turned inward responds very well to counseling and lifestyle changes.

It's important to clarify that the term *depression* as discussed in this chapter is not necessarily a deep and profound clinical depression. Rather, it could range from feeling down in the dumps, sad, or hopeless from time to time to being a much deeper clinical depression that requires professional intervention. If your depression is so deep that you are unable to function in daily activities like basic hygiene, getting out of bed, or going to work or school, or if you're contemplating suicide, then you must get immediate help from someone qualified to provide that help. Treatment options are effective, numerous, and always improving.

On occasion people do hold onto their depression. You may be wondering why on earth would someone do that, because depression feels awful! Well, we sometimes cling to the thing that's hurting us—depression—because trying to make a change sounds even more painful. Motivation for change typically follows the path of least discomfort. Sometimes it seems impossible to even fathom that there is another, less painful, perspective.

The opposite of depression is not happiness. The opposite of depression is vitality. With vitality, you enjoy health and well-being to the point of joy. Vitality is an awakening of your passions and your purpose in a way that is balanced and energizing. It's a sustained awareness of what lights you up. When you lack vitality, you are more likely to experience symptoms of depression. You can ease this by clarifying where to set boundaries so that you can align with your vitality. Ultimately, the journey is more valuable than the destination. Find out what moves you, and go do it.

GET MOVING TO BOOST MOOD

When you have MDD or PDD, it may feel impossible or even insulting to hear that you should exercise. But these suggestions are not intended to insult you or to diminish the challenge that your depression presents. I suggest exercise because I strongly believe that exercise will help. And so the goal is to figure out a way to make that happen. Depression can cause actual physical pain and extreme fatigue. It can feel very difficult to even entertain the idea of exercise. I think it's important to create an open space for every woman to define exercise in the way that works for her. Progress comes from consistency. Baby steps are still steps, and no starting point is too modest. It's all good as long as it feels good to you.

If you're suffering from depression, getting dressed and going outside can feel like a Herculean task. It is not necessary to go to the gym if that feels insurmountable. Home workouts, yoga, and walking around your neighborhood are all beneficial. Start where you are. Resist the urge to compare yourself to anyone else. If you have depression, the goal is to nurture yourself every moment of every day. The worst thing you can do with depression is either act like it's not there or let it define you. You are not your depression.

Getting started with exercise when you have depression is different from dealing with any other physical limitation. More than any other time in your life when you're trying to fit exercise into a busy schedule, exercise for a sufferer of depression has to be simple and accessible. If you struggle with thoughts of self-harm and anger toward your body, you may be tempted to push exercise to the point of pain. This is counterproductive and dangerous and should serve as a red flag that you need to get additional support.

Exercise can be the ideal starting point for healing feelings of hopelessness or inadequacy if you can stay committed to only doing exercise that is nurturing and leaves you filled with a sense of self-respect for where you are in this moment. Blending yoga with a walking program is one approach, but it's important that you choose what speaks to you. Exercise should never hurt, even if—*especially if*—you have depression. If you have depression *and* PCOS, you're hurting enough already.

From a neurological standpoint, the causes of depression are similar to the causes of anxiety. In general, people who have depression have reduced levels of serotonin, the feel-good chemical. However, different factors affect the likelihood of depression occurring, including genetics, changes in hormone levels, medications, stress, or persistent sadness.

There is an association between depression and insulin resistance.[7] If you have PCOS and you're seeing a psychiatrist for depression, you will definitely want to inform her of your diagnosis and of any medications you might be taking for your PCOS. For many women who suffer from both PCOS and depression, reversing the high testosterone and insulin resistance has been enough to resolve the depression. It has been shown that the physical symptoms of PCOS alone aren't always the cause of depression. Depression has been shown to be linked to insulin resistance partly because people who have depression have a tendency to eat more sugar, drink more alcohol, exercise less, and sleep more than necessary, which contributes to insulin resistance. Insulin can affect serotonin levels, so if you have depression, a healthy lifestyle can aid in your recovery.

Any medications that decrease insulin resistance, such as spironolactone and metformin, could potentially have mood-boosting benefits for women with PCOS. If you have been struggling with depression for any length of time, I recommend that you also work with a counselor to become aware of habits or ingrained thinking patterns that might slow your recovery.

Insulin has been found to promote tryptophan availability to the brain. As a result, it can be guessed that drugs that improve insulin sensitivity might also be useful in treating depression for women who have PCOS.

The good news is that if depression is linked to PCOS, then treating PCOS can help resolve the depression in the first six weeks, even if it takes up to six months to resolve the physical symptoms.[8]

Clinical diagnoses aside, more often than not, when a client comes to me and tells me she is depressed, she is mild to moderately depressed. She's feeling sad, down in the dumps, bummed. Maybe it's been going on for some time and is related to a certain event or life change. In these cases, we carefully consider the need for medical and psychological intervention. If clinical care is not necessary, or if it is necessary and in place, our first approach from a lifestyle perspective is going to be exercise.

Just ten minutes of exercise a day is enough to reverse the flow of energy and provides a safe way to ease back into daily life with more energy, a more positive outlook, and, with continued exercise, an emotional resilience that is hard to produce any other way.

If you want to try exercise to ease depression, then consider these options:

Commit to ten minutes of exercise a day—Many fitness plans come with built-in rest days, but if you're exercising to cope with or reduce depression, the ideal is to exercise for at least ten minutes a day, every day. You may have to scale back the intensity of the exercise to be able to sustain it healthily, but daily exercise is ideal to both ease symptoms of depression and maintain long-term motivation!

Start simply—If you're suffering with depression, making a big change in your lifestyle might feel overwhelming. No need to go to extremes! Walking is a wonderful exercise—it's simple, portable, uncomplicated, and low cost, and you can adjust the time spent and intensity to suit your needs. But walking is just a suggestion; I recommend that you pick any exercise that sparks your interest.

Respect your limits, but have faith in your abilities—You are not a machine. You will have good days and bad days, and that is completely normal. Respect yourself enough to burn off the excess energy, but make sure to do so without bullying yourself. Discuss any concerns with your doctor or counselor.

Get medical clearance before undertaking an exercise program—Talk to your doctor to make sure you are physically healthy enough to do the exercise you are planning to do. If there is any doubt or concern about your physical ability, it can inhibit motivation. Once you know that you are physically ready for exercise, it becomes easier to separate physical fatigue from the symptoms of depression.

Start small—Choose incredibly small, achievable goals where you can build on your success. There are hundreds of free downloadable fitness apps with exercise plans that are progressive, building on the previous day's success. If you start out on day one trying to do a hundred squats, you're probably going to hurt yourself, and your chances of staying with it are slim. By starting with small, simple goals and building progressively, you learn how to incorporate this new routine into your life, which cuts down on a lot of emotional resistance.

Think about what you want from your exercise time—Do you need more time for yourself, or do you feel lonely and want a workout buddy?

Your exercise time is yours to shape in any way that meets your needs.
If you have depression and want to work out with a partner, make sure
you work out with someone who understands your depression and is
willing to be your cheerleader (without being completely annoying).

Keep it private for now—Don't share your new exercise plans with your
Facebook friends or family, thinking that it will keep you accountable
later on. Talking about your plans sets you up for feelings of shame
if you happen to struggle to achieve them. You don't need that if
you're already treating depression. Exercise is something you do for
yourself, not anyone else. Keeping it to yourself keeps your motivation coming from within.

Talk to your family about the time you need for exercise—This is different from talking about your exercise plans. If your family is used to
having your attention at any given moment, this may be hard. Resist
the urge to ask for permission in any way. You don't need permission
to take care of yourself. Give them advance notice, and stick to your
schedule as much as possible. Sure, situations may come up where
you can't stick to your plan, but as this will be a learning experience
for your family, keep in mind that sticking to the plan will help them
adjust to your new routine so that you don't have to expend a huge
amount of emotional energy every time you try to get out the door.

Regular exercise can protect you from future struggles with depression.
When you are exercising regularly, you are maintaining the flow of energy
outward and maintaining balance. Also, you are building self-esteem from
a series of small successes—from completing a daily exercise routine. And
self-esteem will give you a *healthy* sense of outrage if your life starts to
take another difficult turn.

The research is still undecided as to whether exercise will *cure* depression. However, I believe that even if exercise is not a cure, it loosens the
rigid thought processes that keep people stuck in depression and allows for
a different perspective to emerge.

Another way exercise can improve depression is to serve as a foundation
that one can then build upon. For example, if you're feeling overwhelmed
with work, life, and other responsibilities, the power of choosing to care for
yourself, if only for ten minutes a day, cannot be overstated. Breathe, take
a step, and breathe again. Repeat this for ten minutes a day (or longer!),
and you will begin to see that you can make similar progress in other parts
of your life. I often tell clients that consistency beats intensity. Nothing

could be more true than when using exercise to treat depression. Choose something you can do every day, even on your worst day, and do it consistently. Then watch as the depression lifts like a heavy fog and you gain momentum toward your goals. That said, if exercise feels impossible, it's important to be gentle with yourself. Don't bully yourself into exercising if the depression is too heavy. The most important thing is to ask for help when you need it and to do what's best for you. Daily affirmations, meditation, and even sitting outside on a pretty day with a cup of tea are all ideas that will help boost your mood.

LONG-TERM MANAGEMENT OF DEPRESSION

If you have had depression once and have recovered, the risk of relapse is 50 percent. The chances of relapse increase each time there is a recurrence.[9] For women with PCOS, the trigger for relapse into depression can be getting off track with diet and exercise or discontinuing medication, resulting in an increase in insulin resistance. Diligent management is essential for both your health and your emotional well-being.

Other triggers for depression relapse include ruminating, which means repeatedly beating yourself up over every perceived physical and character flaw. Whether the criticism is coming from you or someone else doesn't matter. Criticism lowers your energy and mind-set for virtually every aspect of your life. Energy works with a sort of momentum: what you put energy toward will continue, for better or worse.

Another cause of relapse into depression is not knowing what your triggers are. This is one area where mindfulness can help tremendously. To avoid this type of relapse, look at past episodes with depression. What stands out as a trigger? Are there any dates on the calendar that upset you? This could be the anniversary of a loss of some sort or an upcoming event that you dread.

What sorts of responsibilities do you have during the day? If you wear a variety of hats, then you know it's important to consider them separately. What about your job drains you emotionally? Do you feel stuck in a hopeless relationship? Not only does this simplify introspection, but it also serves as a natural reminder that nothing is all good or all bad.

Relapse can also be prevented by eating plenty of nutritious food. Avoid sugars and alcohol. Many of the foods containing tryptophan that help with anxiety also help with depression.

Express anger in a way that is effective and safe. Journaling is enormously helpful for this. If you struggle with managing or expressing anger, talking to a therapist can be enormously helpful.

Maintain a regular sleep schedule. While it may seem fun to stay up late and binge-watch your favorite TV series, you're likely to feel tired the next day. If you're tired the next day, you're likely to make poor health decisions the next day, like oversleeping and missing the gym. If you're tired, it can feel difficult to elevate your thoughts. Elevated thoughts will keep you from ruminating.

Avoid loneliness by choosing to surround yourself with people you love and trust. Quantity does not equal quality. Superficial relationships can be a distraction but are not nearly as helpful as connecting with people who really care about you. Real connections matter because they are what will actually help you when the going gets tough.

Whether you're going through your first round of depression or you've done this a few times, or your depression has never reached clinical levels but you want to shake off the blues, the best thing you can do is respond as soon as you know that you're heading in that direction. Don't wait for your symptoms to worsen before you make positive changes and ask for help.

If depression is interfering with any of your functioning, seek the help of a professional trained in depression. Start with your regular doctor, find a therapist you like, and seek the counsel of a psychiatrist if medication is recommended. Depression can be addressed and controlled, but you don't have to do it on your own. It can also be devastating. But it does not have to be something you suffer alone. Take the first step. It may be hard, but it may lead down a rewarding path.

JOURNAL QUESTIONS

1. What problem or worry keeps coming back into your mind?
2. What are you grateful for? In fact, I recommend that you keep a daily gratitude journal.
3. What advice would you give to another woman suffering from depression?
4. What are you feeling when you feel depressed? Give a name to those emotions.

7

Self-Esteem, Self-Care, Self-Worth

When you are first diagnosed with PCOS, it may be tempting to go through a "why me?" period. Grieve the loss of what you thought your body should do. Then get excited about the small wins you are going to create every day.

Imagine going from feeling depressed, dismayed, and wondering, *What is my body doing?* to feeling exhilarated and marveling, *Look what my body can do!* That's the purpose of a lifestyle strategy for better health. Self-care is the behavioral result of self-esteem; however, it is possible to fake it 'til you make it and then gradually build self-esteem with a commitment to self-care activities.

SELF-ESTEEM

Whether it is a mild concern about irregular periods or deep, heart-wrenching disappointment over potential issues with infertility, PCOS can chip away at your self-esteem. It's important to be aware of the way low self-esteem can impact all areas of your life.

Where do you feel inadequate? Like you're not enough? Is it coming from that voice in your head, or have you gotten direct criticism from other people in your life?

Whatever the case, let me just stop right here. You *are* worthy of self-care. You *are* special, unique, and amazing. Be very careful not to define yourself by the insensitive remarks of others. The truth is that they likely do not understand your health issues and may think they are being helpful.

Comments may sting, but they are often born of ignorance rather than malice. Still, struggling with any health issue can do a number on a person's self-esteem. We often measure ourselves by expectations we think others have for us. The truth is more likely that others don't think of us nearly as often as we think they do. In this chapter, I'm going to show you how to get self-esteem back.

You may be thinking, *That's great, but I can't just forget about hurtful criticism.* Maybe not, but you *can* choose how you receive it. When you receive a message that may wear away at your self-esteem or block your attempts at self-care, try to remember to stop and ask yourself, *What is the underlying message here?* Even better, ask yourself, *What is the feeling behind what is being said?*

Many women try to compensate for their PCOS by being perfect in other areas of life. While it is positive to give energy to what you can change instead of what you can't, the quest for perfection is not helpful and can only serve to erode your self-esteem. The path to perfection is paved with negative self-talk. What's worse, perfection is a mirage. You never get to "perfect."

Most people with low self-esteem believe that they have to wait until they reach a certain goal before feeling like they deserve a positive self-assessment. The truth is that the right to love yourself and take care of yourself accordingly is undeniable.

How to Boost Your Self-Esteem while Achieving Your Goals

The first step toward healthy self-esteem is to understand that there is nothing wrong with where you are now. It is simply your starting point. Release any self-criticism, and appreciate that you have clarity about your starting point.

Now, set a goal, and then backtrack to create a path to your starting point. Don't just think about it. Write it down and tack it to your wall. If you get stuck going from one goal to the next, it's okay to spend more time in one stage—or, better yet, break down that step into even smaller steps so that it feels more attainable.

Every Day Do Something—Anything—Connected with Your Goal

Keep your reasons for healthy lifestyle change in the forefront of your mind while you go through this. Ending the war with yourself and healing the relationship might take some time. If you can't fathom making changes for yourself, try making changes for something you love, something you feel deep down in your core. This is a valid and worthy stand-in until that happens. It's a slightly different route that gets you to the same place: self-love, self-esteem, and self-respect.

Finding Your Why

Why you are working on yourself is powerful and can make or break your efforts for healthy lifestyle change. The biggest mistake *most* people make is that they don't get deep enough with their why. Many gurus will tell you, *Your why should make you cry*, and there is truth to it beyond the fact that it rhymes and sounds good. The important part of getting deep on your why is so that you can get past the thought processes (and the superficial stories we make up about ourselves) and into the feelings part of our experience. This is because the behavioral response to feelings is much more powerful and efficient than our response to thoughts. Thoughts are malleable. We can think our way into and out of anything. Our response to feelings, on the other hand, is essentially automatic. Bottom line: gut reactions will get you to the gym long before reasoning will.

If you lose motivation, chances are that the jump from one step to another is too great. Break it down even further. There is no shame in taking baby steps. This is your journey, and there is every reason to celebrate any degree of progress. Occasionally look back and see how far you've come—not just in numbers on the scale but also in all the times you chose to exercise and eat right when you could have chosen not to.

One of the biggest self-esteem traps for women with PCOS is to compare herself to other women. You may be tempted to hold onto this because there may be truth to it. Yes, there are other women who don't struggle with insulin resistance, or infertility, but that doesn't make them better or more successful than you. Comparing yourself is a tremendous waste of energy because we all have different paths, different challenges, and different work to do. Their path is their path. Your path is yours. Take that energy you've been wasting on comparing yourself to others and apply it to the work you are doing now.

The comparison trap you lay for yourself may be difficult to bypass because it has been carefully constructed along a well-worn path. And so it will take practice to disrupt this pattern, but this work is as important as reducing insulin resistance. Just as PCOS has far-reaching effects on your body and moods, self-esteem has far-reaching effects on the way you treat your body. As such, self-esteem serves as a powerful platform to making positive changes in your health and well-being.

It's important to monitor and describe emotional pain when our culture seems to value the self-contained approach. Just as children learn to care for minor wounds, they need to learn to care for emotional wounds large and small. Some emotional injuries are inevitable, but we have the power to choose how we react to them. Protect and nurture your self-esteem at all costs.

I combined self-esteem and self-care in the same chapter because they are connected. The more self-esteem you have, the more you are able to make self-care a priority.

The opposite is also true. If your self-esteem decreases, it makes effective, efficient self-care hard to fathom. Some people prefer a fake-it-'til-you-make-it approach. If you can commit to self-care even if you don't feel worthy, you will begin to feel more empowered and have an improved opinion of yourself. This may mean committing to a weekly massage, a daily run, or going to the gym regularly. Progress, not perfection, is the essence of lasting lifestyle change.

Self-esteem is described by Dr. Guy Winch as the emotional immune system.[1] Without it, we are more susceptible to anxiety, depression, and dysfunctional relationships. But it can get even worse: Low self-esteem can lead to more physical health problems. It can make it harder to make positive choices to take care of yourself in the way you eat and exercise. It can make it harder for you to stick up for yourself when there are too many demands on your time and energy.

Self-esteem is not an all-or-nothing feeling. Like any diet or fitness endeavor, it must be maintained. There are some red flags that indicate your self-esteem could use extra attention. Examples include feeling depressed. Perhaps this has been going on so long it has turned into clinical depression. You might find yourself feeling discouraged, feeling like things won't turn out well, or perhaps you worry about being rejected.

We see this a lot in relationships. Do you let others set the boundaries in the relationship? Perhaps it is because you worry about their opinion of you or you don't trust your instincts. You may come across as confident and smart, but if you have low self-esteem, then you have chinks in the armor that narcissistic bullies pick up on. This can leave you more vulnerable to a chaotic or even abusive relationship. Women with low self-esteem also tend to be more sensitive within relationships, which can weigh a relationship down.

Working women also sometimes struggle to feel like they are worthy of a promotion, or they lack the confidence to speak up in a meeting, even if they know their contribution is both relevant and useful.

People with low self-esteem might find themselves overly concerned about the opinions of others. This is a fear that can limit personal growth. You might worry about what people say about your college major or how you prefer to dress. You might worry about how people will see you at the gym, making it harder to find the motivation to go. And as a result of your low self-esteem, it becomes almost impossible to live with passion and purpose.

If you have low self-esteem, you might tend to make mountains out of molehills. If you say something awkward at the checkout line, you might spend a lot of time beating yourself up for it later. And this can easily develop into ruminating over the event, which can then create a criticism-paved path to depression. Rumination is a trigger for depression. If you give in to that downward spiral of negative thinking, it only gets worse, which can send you into something quite negative. Thoughts are controllable if you catch them before they become an addiction. When you find yourself ruminating, you can *decide* to think about something positive. With practice, it's a mind-set shift that is nearly automatic and applicable to every part of your life.

Strategies to Elevate Self-Esteem

To start building up your self-esteem, try on the following suggestions:

Avoid "should" statements—Whenever you say you "should" do something, there's an implied criticism, as if to say, *How dare you do it any other way?* Criticism is poison to relationships. Self-esteem is all about enhancing the relationship you have with yourself. Ease up on the should, and eliminate self-criticism to elevate self-esteem.

Avoid overgeneralizing—Are there things you say that you "always" or "never" do? Have you really taken a look at whether that is true? Do you have proof to back up your belief? For example, if you have an awkward moment with a new date, try to avoid beating yourself up and applying the "awkward" label to all future dates. Can you remember a time when a first date went really well?

Be intentional with your thoughts—Notice any patterns in your thoughts that don't serve you well, and decide to consider a different perspective.[2] It might take some energy to be more aware of these exceptions to long-held beliefs. Journaling about this topic can be enormously helpful.

Appreciate your PCOS—How do your PCOS or your ways of coping with PCOS become a positive thing? Your first impulse might be to say, *Nothing!* The truth is that, while your symptoms might be under control, the syndrome will always be there. Fighting something that you cannot change is not an efficient way to use your energy. Try something new. Call a truce, and look for something positive. You may find that your body builds muscle more easily than other women. You might know more about your body and how to nourish it with the proper foods. You might love the process of getting healthy and giving other women with PCOS hope and inspiration.

Decide how you like your eggs (and more!)—So many women have no idea what makes them happy or fulfilled. Perhaps they were told long ago that their ideas were foolish or selfish. Perhaps no one even asked. Whatever the case may be, now is the time to think it through. What do you like for breakfast? What is your favorite TV show? Coffee or tea? Get your journal out, and decide what you like about everything you can think of. No preference is too mundane or insignificant. Getting clear on what you like is the first (and most powerful) step to actually getting it.

Help someone—Consider volunteering or tutoring. You might choose to volunteer in a way that is in keeping with your strengths (for example, if you're good with computers, you might help a homeless shelter with their website, or if you're good at math, you might tutor in an after-school program). Or perhaps volunteering in something that is entirely outside of your routine could become a breath of fresh air.

SELF-CARE

Are you the strong one? The one who makes things happen? The one everyone looks to when it's time to get things done?

If so, then I want to know: Who is taking care of you?

If you're struggling to take care of your PCOS, then I can bet you have needs that aren't being met. Notice I didn't say *wants*. Unmet wants don't necessarily have consequences when they are left unmet. We're talking about needs. This is an important distinction, because your body has probably let you get away with a lot but, when your needs aren't being met, there's an adjustment or correction somewhere else—often in the form of a symptom. If you've been neglecting yourself and haven't yet suffered any consequences from it, consider yourself lucky, because *yet* is the key word here.

Most people think that self-care is all about grand gestures, but, done well, it's all in the details woven in throughout your day. It takes energy to practice emotional self-care. At times proper self-care can feel like an investment made on blind faith. Self-care isn't an all-or-nothing endeavor. Instead, it is possible (and incredibly useful) to nudge the dial back toward yourself just a bit.

Just Do It

Whatever your self-care activities are, make sure they are personally rewarding. Don't do something you hate just because someone else found it to be helpful. Our culture has placed self-care in the "negotiable" category—the first thing to go when we don't have time to get everything done. And so often this tendency is exacerbated by guilt when we are asked to help others, even when we're overcommitted.

The fact is that self-care is nonnegotiable. When we don't do it, our bodies and minds compensate—and it's not healthy. For clarity, self-care should look to both physical self-care and emotional self-care. I also highly recommend spiritual self-care.

Physical self-care might be getting enough sleep or making sure that you stay hydrated, getting daily exercise, and eating foods that are good for your body.

Mental self-care includes mental hygiene. Just like we know how to care for a minor cut, we need to learn how to handle minor emotional events so that they heal well. How do you handle rejection? How do you cope with grief? Toughing it out by telling yourself that "time heals all wounds" isn't enough. To be happy and healthy, you have to take action to care for your mental health.

The idea of emotional hygiene was presented by Dr. Guy Winch in a TED Talk.[3] He made the case that emotional hygiene has a profound effect on mental and physical health and that, as a community, we are choosing a mindless routine over a sense of connectedness and well-being.

Accept and acknowledge your feelings. Too many women are made to feel temperamental or silly for expressing emotions, but nothing could be further from the truth. Identify, acknowledge, and accept your emotions. Release the need to put a value on them. Feelings are neither good nor bad. They are there to help us make sense of what we are experiencing. If you struggle to identify your feelings, it can help to go through a list of emotions and journal about whatever comes up. Are your angry or enraged? Are you sad or crushed? The nuances matter when you're trying to gain insight. Try an Internet search to fill your list of possible emotions you want to consider.

Change the scenery. You could take an afternoon off and go to the beach, or you could simply go outside for a change of sensory experience. For example, when you are feeling down or even just lazy you might go outside and feel the grass between your toes, or you might do some deep breathing or get a massage.

If your family, friends, and work don't meet your needs, no problem, no hard feelings; it simply means that it's time for you to take care of you. The nice thing about self-care is that it's the most efficient kind of care you can receive. No one knows what you want or need more than you.

Are you fine, or are you *fulfilled*? There is fulfilled, and there is fine. Most of us make the mistake of being merely fine. Don't be fine. Fine is unfulfilled. That creates a gap that is usually managed with unhealthy coping strategies. The closer you can get to fulfilled, the easier it becomes to make healthier choices for yourself with more consistency.

Making Self-Care Happen

The question, very often, is *Where do I even start?*

Start where you are, not where you think you should be. Change should be slow—so slow that you wonder if it's working but feel giddy over how easy it feels. That second part is crucial. Most women who have PCOS and obesity have spent years fighting with their bodies. If asked, they can give a detailed list of what their bodies can't do.

The first goal of exercise is to redefine that perspective. Take the list of what your body can't do, and toss it out of the window. Even if the list seems accurate, it's not helping in the least, and it's time to unplug the energy source powering it. The time has come to make a list of what your body can do, and exercise is the place to start.

Start simply. You can always increase the intensity later on, but if you do too much too soon, you'll quickly burn out—or, worse, injure yourself. When starting an exercise routine, stop before feeling fatigued. You're looking for that motivational sweet spot that will serve you well when it comes to making exercise a daily part of life. Your goal may not be to lose weight, but it is to gain health. The reality is that once you reach your goal weight, you still have to keep going. Start the way you mean to go on—not in intensity but in the way you want to feel about exercise. The definition of ideal exercise will naturally vary from one person to the next; however, there are guidelines that will transform exercise into lasting lifestyle change.

Self-care is easier said than done. A helpful tip? Remember why you started. This is your long-term health that we are talking about. There is no perfect time to start, no perfect day. Your motivation is only as strong as your worst day, so that is actually an excellent starting point. Don't hesitate; just begin, and stay open to working out the details as you go along.

When it comes to self-care, it can be helpful to put your focus on what self-care activities will give you the greatest return on your investment of time and energy. For example, sitting and watching TV for thirty minutes is fairly relaxing, but thirty minutes of exercise is rejuvenating. You're not just looking to take the pressure off; you're also looking to recharge. Consistency will intensify this effect. What sorts of things rebuild your body and mind? Make a list of your top ten, and next to each indicate how long it takes to complete that activity. Then put them in order of how rejuvenating they are. Keep that list handy, and look it over any time you're feeling overwhelmed or exhausted.

Here are some ideas for healthy rebuilding:

exercise (running, walking, swimming, biking, weight training)
reading
massage
having your hair done
meditation
yoga/stretching
playing a board game with family and friends
preparing your lunches for the week
saying no to something you don't want to do
enjoying a cup of hot tea or lemon water

Avoid these empty activities:

scanning social media
watching too much TV without purpose
playing video games
mindless eating
excessive alcohol consumption
spending time with toxic friends
spending too much time in worry, self-criticism, or resentment
making something perfect
repeatedly having the same argument with a loved one

Keep in mind that, when you're exhausted at the end of the day, it's likely not that you're physically exhausted but mentally exhausted, so it's worth looking for ways to boost your mental energy and reduce stress. The goal is to balance burning off physical energy with boosting mental energy so that you are at your peak performance.

Tips for Dealing with Close Family and Friends

When it comes to self-care, it can be hard to change the status quo. This is especially true when you have a family or significant other. We naturally want to maintain the status quo in our relationships, because it takes so much energy to alter an established pattern. Our loved ones have expectations of us, and it can feel like a failure when we don't meet those expectations.

To help your family cope with your changing lifestyle, make slow and steady changes. This is helpful because most people can tolerate being inconvenienced for a short time. With consistency, though, the inconvenience turns to adaptation with the least amount of resistance. Consistency also helps you stay on track with your goals.

Give lots of warning ahead of time. This is a tricky one. On one hand, you don't want to set yourself up for feelings of failure or shame if you don't follow through, but if there is a new change to your activities or schedule that you're sure is going to happen, it is easier to give a lot of warning so others can adjust—or at the very least can't be mad because you gave them fair warning. You may even consider including your significant others in your exercise routines. Perhaps you plan to walk once a day, whether it's in the morning before work or after dinner. Include a friend or partner. Walking and talking can be a great way to strengthen a relationship while also getting some much-needed exercise and fresh air.

Self-Defeating Behavior

Just as we should brainstorm for ways to build ourselves up, we should also be vigilant about ways we tear ourselves down. Consider the following examples:

- You're seeing results on the scale.
  - o *Sabotage*—When you lose weight, it's not just your clothing size that changes. You may also feel an increased sense of personal power. People might see you differently (it's not fair, but it's often the reality). Your role in your inner circle may change. Even your relationship with your spouse can change. Changing roles can be painful and scary, even if totally normal, so many people fall back into familiar patterns, resulting in regaining the weight they lost.
  - o *How to work though it*—Be mindful. Be aware that this dynamic can exist. When fear or resistance set in, you don't have to solve it; just acknowledge it without judgment. Remind yourself why you're losing weight, and stay focused. Remember, this is a process, and it's better to take it slowly so that everyone (including yourself) has a chance to adjust to the results you're getting.
- You're losing weight for the wrong reasons.
  - o *Sabotage*—If you lose weight so that hot guy will like you, so you can get the job of your dreams, or so you can be the popular girl, then you may be disappointed and revert back to old patterns when those goals don't materialize.
  - o *How to work through it*—The goal of weight loss is better physical and emotional health. Yes, it's nice to have your clothes fit better, but be careful not to hinge your efforts on secondary motivators.
- You eat to reward yourself for working out.
  - o *Sabotage*—This is so easy to do. You worked hard in that kickboxing class. Surely that's worth a pizza and beer, right? The problem is that we tend to overestimate calorie burn and underestimate calories consumed.
  - o *How to work through it*—Use a food-tracking app like My Fitness Pal. Yes, adherence will take getting used to, but it's entirely worth it, as you can get real about your calorie budget.

Body Image

Body image refers to the way you view yourself, but the effects of body image fan out into every part of our experience. It's the way you meet the world and has a huge impact on the way the world meets you in return. Body image is a large part of what makes up self-esteem. Like other aspects of health, body image is not a destination but a journey that calls for balance, awareness, and effort.

While body image is your judgment of your looks, self-esteem is the judgment you assign to who you are as a person. Self-esteem isn't all-or-nothing; it's not good or bad. It's even hard to define it as being either high or low. Many people will find that in some situations their self-esteem is positive, whereas in other areas it's much more negative. However, if you find that your self-esteem is consistently lower, then it's time for a reboot.

When asked what they think about their bodies, many women—especially women with PCOS—have a list of things they want to change that is much longer than the list of things they like. It's possible to love yourself exactly as you are and still want better for it. In fact, this is the balance that you will have to find in order to make the most consistent, positive changes for yourself. Obviously, if it were as simple as deciding to change your mind-set, then we'd all have fantastic self-esteem and amazing body image. Unfortunately, it's not that simple. The solution for low self-esteem and distorted body image starts with self-compassion; however, women with PCOS very often struggle with this because our bodies are not doing what we want them to do.

When you are frustrated with your body, it can be easy to lose touch with it and even lose respect for it, which creates a self-defeating cycle that can be tough to break. It's important to give focus to this. The way we treat ourselves becomes the blueprint for the way others will treat us. While it's never excusable for someone to hurt or insult you, there exists within you a power that is likely not turned on, which then makes you more vulnerable to emotional or even physical harm.

When self-esteem is low and body image is negative, it's like a smoke alarm that has been set too far away from the kitchen. It takes a lot more negativity to raise the internal alarm, to find our sense of healthy outrage that says, *This is not okay*. Just because you can endure something doesn't mean that it's right. The time has come to put health and self-awareness together. For women with PCOS, it's important that we get this sooner rather than later. Women are usually much better at criticizing their bodies than affirming their bodies. Usually my clients can make a list of personal criticisms so specific and thorough that even they would see it as hatefully nitpicky if the same appraisal were applied to their friends.

The reason that body image is so hard to change is because it is supported by a tremendous infrastructure of stories—or, more specifically, histories, as these messages have often been in place for a long time. The problem, however, is that the story has about as much basis in fact as our people-watching skills at the airport. Sitting at your gate, watching the swarms of strangers passing, your mind can come up with a complete story for each of them, including motivations, insecurities, and personal preferences. While this is an entertaining time-killer until boarding time, when you apply this kind of definition to yourself, it creates a fixed mindset that makes behavior change difficult. It's like driving a car and getting stuck in the mud.

For women with PCOS, the list of self-critique generally targets our femininity, fertility, and fitness—areas that impact the very essence of being a woman and hit where we feel most vulnerable and most out of control. The problem with this is that it naturally leads to a fixed mind-set, making even the idea of a healthy lifestyle change seem inconceivable. Further, many women have such depleted self-esteem that they are left doubting whether they even deserve the effort it takes to make healthy lifestyle changes.

Redefining your body image isn't a one-and-done activity. It's not a destination. The most confident and self-assured people have made a habit · of creating useful thought patterns. More simply, they have redefined the stories they tell about themselves into something that supports healthy lifestyle changes.

The best way to start this process is to make up a new story. You may be thinking, *You want me to lie?* Absolutely not. What I want you to do is ignore your perceived weakness for now and instead give all of your energy to your strengths. If you're struggling with this activity, consider how your friends would describe you. What are your positive characteristics?

Focus on the Positive

Have you ever worked with a personal trainer at the gym? The shoddy ones identify your weak points and attempt to strengthen them, but what ends up happening is that you feel uncoordinated and hurt for days afterward. There is no motivation in the world that can put up with that. What's worse is that we pay for it! Unfortunately, it plays right into the low self-esteem that many of us carry into the gym. The underlying message is that you have to get to a certain (random) point of ability before you can gain approval. The truth is that your mind won't put up with that emotional and physical pain for long. Build your body image by giving energy to your strengths.

Recovering from PCOS is not a series of hoops you jump through to get to a destination. It's an all-encompassing lifestyle change, so doing it right takes time. The good news is that doing it right feels empowering and exciting.

Make a list of all the things you love about your body. Do you have powerful legs? Can you crush the free weights? Maybe you enjoy walking. Wherever it is, start where you are. Embrace what you love. You will find that it expands the more attention you give it.

Healing and strengthening your body image doesn't just happen in your mind; it is a process that can be nurtured by your behavior. Another way to loosen the bonds of negative body image is to play with body language. I say *play* because we tend to get stuck in one way of interacting and so it can be refreshing to try a different approach. For example, if your story is that you're shy and you're at a dinner party with your arms crossed, what would it be like to loosen your arms and take on a more open stance? The goal is not to be inauthentic but to guess and check: Are you shy because you're really shy, or are you shy because that's a story you've told yourself? The same thing applies to your body: Do you avoid caring for yourself because you have no other choice, or do you avoid caring for yourself because tolerating disappointment is the expectation you've established with yourself when it comes to PCOS?

Redefining the Story of You

So, we need to change the story. First, become aware of messages that are feeding your current body image. Images and other messages in the media are common culprits. The problem with these is that they are so common we barely notice them, but the effect is powerful and pervasive. Then ask yourself: Is this message true? Is it kind? Is it permanent?

If you have PCOS, you may be tempted to think that the condition as it is right now is permanent. This fixed mind-set makes sustained motivation feel impossible. If you have PCOS, taking care of your body with an appropriate diet and daily exercise can work wonders to reduce the effects of the condition, but it can also help you create a new story about your body. You will always have PCOS, but the impact it has on your mind and body can evolve over time. For example, you could say, *I have PCOS, so it's impossible to lose weight.* With consistent diet and exercise, that could become *I have PCOS, which I keep in remission with diet and exercise.* Adjusting your perspective changes how you respond to that new perspective, and the results can be dramatic.

Self-Care Strategies for Women with PCOS

When it comes to self-care, simple is better. Sure, elaborate bubble baths and mani-pedis at your favorite spa are divine and can certainly recharge you; however, for most of us the investment of time and money makes that kind of pampering a luxury. The truth is that self-care should be as non-negotiable as taking a shower.

Make a list of things that nurture you in body, mind, or spirit that take thirty seconds or less to complete. Then choose three or four to incorporate into your day, every day.

Need some suggestions?

Drink a glass of water—Staying well hydrated can reduce cravings. Buy a water bottle you love, and make it a habit to keep it with you. Some people will drink more water when they fill and empty small glasses throughout the day; if that is more like you, acknowledge it, and keep a cup of water nearby at all times.

Pray—If you're spiritual, this is an option that has the potential to reduce feelings of hopelessness, anxiety, and isolation. The wonderful thing about prayer is that it can be done anytime and anywhere.

Stretch—No need to make time for a lengthy yoga session. A gentle stretch is a wonderful way to release tense muscles and can give you an emotional boost in the process.

Think about your Big Reason Why—Ultimately, your reason why is motivating. Even if it makes you cry or makes you angry, it gives you purpose and direction. Honor that feeling by taking one small step toward your goals.

Go outside for some fresh air—Fresh air and sunshine can give you a fresh perspective and stimulate creative problem solving. Open the curtains on sunny days. Let natural light into your indoor space.

If you have a pet, cuddle with them for a while—This can reduce blood pressure and can ease emotional pain.

Say something nice to someone else—Sending out positive vibes is a surefire way to boost your mood.

Improve your space—Don't get overwhelmed. Sometimes just taking out the trash or getting all of the half-empty water bottles out of your car is all you can do for now, and that's actually enough to make you feel lighter, clearer, and more together.

Self-care is essential for women with PCOS for a few reasons:

Chronic conditions are hard—You don't get to walk away from PCOS. That's a lot to deal with emotionally! You must go above and beyond so that you ensure you get the recharging your body and mind need so that you can keep a positive mind-set.

We are our own worst critic—Elevating your perspective is essential for maintaining healthy habits.

Stress makes PCOS worse—Stress creates cortisol, and cortisol fights insulin, which creates insulin resistance. Managing stress is more than a mental-health strategy; it's a physical-health strategy too.

SELF-WORTH AND SELF-CARE

When it comes to your list of priorities, where do *you* fall on the list? One mistake that many women with PCOS make is to make decisions about how much love and attention their body *deserves*.

As women with PCOS, our bodies are different, not defective. If you are spending your time and energy defining all the ways your body isn't working, then chances are good that you'll stay stuck. This is where a growth mind-set is crucial. You have to believe that you deserve to be healthy. You have to believe you are worth the time and energy to be healthy. Taking care of others at the expense of your health is not acceptable.

Don't play quid pro quo with your body. It doesn't have to give you anything first to deserve being well taken care of. If anything, our bodies deserve extra care because of more specific dietary needs, increased physical reactions to stress, and higher chances of heart disease and diabetes. That doesn't make you weak; it merely defines the best way to take care of yourself.

While having a diagnosis is helpful, it can keep you stuck if you overly define yourself by that diagnosis. You *have* PCOS—*you* are not PCOS. Perhaps you have fat, but you are not fat; you have fingernails, but you are not fingernails. I see this a lot with patients who have anxiety. They tend to make the mistake of overly identifying with that anxiety and as a result find more and more reasons to be anxious. Similarly, women with PCOS tend to spend so much time fighting the PCOS and learning about the causes, symptoms, and treatments that we forget that there could be a time when the PCOS symptoms are completely under control.

What would it look like to be symptom-free? Imagine a woman who's lost one hundred pounds: Her symptoms of PCOS are completely gone. She's even had two healthy pregnancies. What does it feel like to be her? What does she look like? What is she eating? How does she behave? How does she feel about her body?

Many women make the mistake of putting the demands and needs of others before themselves, waiting for permission to be happy. The truth is that you almost never get permission. But the even greater truth is that you don't *need* permission. The time is now to take control of your health.

JOURNAL QUESTIONS

1. What would you like to say to your body? Write it in a letter.
2. How would your best friend describe you?
3. What would you do if you knew you couldn't fail?
4. What are you really good at?
5. How have you taken care of yourself lately?
6. What do you want?

8

Stress

What You Don't Know Can Make You Sick!

God grant me the serenity to accept the things I cannot change, courage
to change the things I can, and wisdom to know the difference.

—Serenity Prayer

Psychologically, stress is bad for everyone; some tolerate it better than
others. However, as a woman with PCOS, your body cannot tolerate
stress well. This is not to say that you are weak or flawed. In fact, by respecting your sensitivity to stress, you are well on your way to a healthier
and happier life compared to your peers who never have a need to examine
the stress they tolerate day after day.

The physical component of stress can be found in the HPA axis. *HPA*
stands for "hypothalamic-pituitary-adrenal," and it is the neuroendocrine
system that is responsible for creating cortisol. In small amounts, cortisol
isn't a bad thing. It is cortisol's job to help the body respond to stressful
events and get back to normal after the stress is over. However, in the case
of chronic stress, an overly stimulated HPA axis has a negative effect on
the immune system, memory, and inflammation.[1]

A stress response is a normal reaction to an abnormal situation. Stressful
events happen, but the reaction to stress can vary from person to person.
For some people, stress has more of a physical effect; for others, the effect
is more emotional. Often, though, it's a combination of the two. Much
of the intensity of stress depends on the person's perception of it, but the

intensity can even depend on the duration and intensity of childhood expo-
sure to stress, which can affect the way the HPA axis is calibrated. I'm not
suggesting that the only way to healthily deal with stress means opening up
a painful past right now—although you might find therapeutic benefit in
addressing it with a counselor. It is important, however, that you know that
stress has a variety of factors. Resist the urge to compare your experience
of stress to others', and don't let anyone bully you into taking on more than
what feels right simply because it isn't stressful to *them*.

Just because you can deal with something doesn't mean you should.
This is the core of the problem with stress and why so many people live
with it. The truth is that there is a release valve on every type of stress; the
trick is to find what works for you.

Notice we are talking about stress *management*, not stress elimination.
Some situations can't be changed, in which case it could take a combination of all approaches to stress management to adequately cope: mental,
physical, long-term, and short-term approaches. The more severe or
complicated the stress, the more intense and thoughtful the management
approach will need to be. Stress is a normal part of life, and dealing with
it is an acquired skill, so be patient with yourself as you learn what works
for you.

COPING WITH STRESS

Yes, and if it is unduly stressful, then it's time to dial it back. Call your
doctor if you have any questions about how your body is reacting to exercise. Exercise should leave you feeling relaxed, not exhausted. Exercise
causes the release of endorphins, one of the body's feel-good chemicals.

Stress affects the body and the mind, so stress-management strategies
must take both into account. For example, a short-term fix for mental stress
might be to repeat a favorite mantra or do some reality checking ("Is what
I'm worried about *really* likely?"). Long-term strategies for coping with
mental stress include daily meditation practice and psychological counseling. To alleviate the effect of stress on the body, you could try stretching,
deep breathing, and wearing more comfortable clothing. Long-term management strategies include daily exercise, getting enough sleep, and eating
nutritious food.

Stress is inflammatory. Many chronically overstressed women end up
with severe bloating in the midsection, achy joints, headaches, and other

physical responses. We have talked about cortisol throughout the book, but it bears repeating because it is incredibly important for women with PCOS to understand the negative impact of cortisol on the body: long-term overexposure to cortisol can have health consequences for anyone, but if you have PCOS, it can be disastrous. Just like a diabetic has to be vigilant about what she eats, you have to be vigilant about stress. It's not fair, but, even so, it's not a sign of weakness. It's simply that, in order to be the healthiest version of yourself, you have to acknowledge this difference and respond accordingly. Stress management is the secret ingredient of any healthy lifestyle change.

Chronic stress occurs because we are conditioned to remove the feeling of stress as quickly as possible without adequately dealing with the stress. The problem with that knee-jerk response is that we don't always choose the healthiest option to relieve the stress. We all have a bag of tricks filled with tools for stress management. For many women, the primary coping strategy is eating, but the quick fix could be anything from shopping to overindulging in alcohol. The better approach to handling stress is to sit with the discomfort for a moment, really take a look at what's causing it, and then decide how to proceed.

You may be wondering why I recommend that you sit with the stress longer. Isn't the point to reduce and relieve stress? Yes, but if you don't really look at it, you won't understand how to actually resolve it, and you are bound to experience that unaddressed stress again with the same level of discomfort. Better to sit with the stressor long enough that you can improve your response to it.

The goal is not to change the stressor; the goal is to change your part in it. Obviously you can't change other people—nor should you try. There are also circumstances like family illnesses or a change in job status that are, to a large degree, very much outside of your control. So focus on the part of the process that is within your control: your response to it.

Most people have a response to stress that is akin to an allergic reaction. But in this case, instead of skyrocketing histamines, it's cortisol levels that overescalate. The body responds to the overabundance of cortisol with inflammation, and that inflammation, over time, can create physical problems like heart disease, joint pain, digestive problems, and even reproductive problems. The digestion and reproductive problems develop because in an immediate threat cortisol reduces nonessential bodily functions in an effort to divert all available energy to the perceived immediate threat. This physiological hyperresponse was useful when we were fighting off saber-toothed tigers, but it isn't as useful when the copy machine is broken, a deadline is looming, and you haven't been to the gym in months.

Granted, stress is a part of life, but much like a fixed budget, you have a finite amount of energy that you can put toward addressing stress before you exceed your healthy limit, so it's important for you to understand where your energy is being drained.

What does it look like to sit with stress? It's looking it in the eye rather than blindly wrestling with it. In choosing to sit with stress, you're not judging yourself or even the stress. You are creating a distance between the event and your understanding of it, through which you can develop awareness of what is unavoidable in a situation, what simply is, and how you choose to react to all of it.

SAYING NO IS YOUR SECRET WEAPON AGAINST STRESS

Some stressors are unavoidable, but when you are pulled in a million different directions and you're feeling overwhelmed, saying no can be a powerful way to manage the kinds of stressors that *are* avoidable. So many women struggle to say no because we have been culturally conditioned to be the relationship builders and the caretakers. Saying no to accepting additional responsibilities, especially when relationships and nurturing are involved, can feel like a personal failure, an attack on the relationship, and like you're letting the other person down. If you struggle with saying no to a telemarketer, then saying no to a friend or family member is infinitely harder. It takes practice to learn how to say no, meaning that you won't get it right every time. And it takes patience—with yourself and with the other people who are used to relying on you to always say yes.

Know Why You're Saying No

Chances are that you're not saying no just to be mean. More likely, you're saying no because saying yes would push you over the edge of giving what you have to give and giving to the point of harm to yourself. For example, you're saying no to the telemarketer because you don't want to spend fifty dollars on a charity you've never heard of. Take time to define the reason you're saying no in other situations, and you may begin to understand and believe that your no is nothing to feel guilty about.

Just because you can say yes in any given moment doesn't mean you should. Respect your limits. When you're in the process of creating a healthy lifestyle, I recommend that you make a habit of buying yourself some time so that you can really think about whether an extra activity is what your body and mind need right now. Daily stress is often made up of many small decisions and activities. You can reduce stress by assessing each of your responsibilities and tasks with a fresh judgment as to whether it's a good fit for the new life you're building.

Different Ways to Say No

So, you've been asked to take on an additional responsibility. You've sat with it. And you've determined that it's best for you to say no. But *how* do you say no? Try one of these responses:

"Not right now."
"Let me think about it." Then send them a firm no via e-mail as soon as possible.
"Sounds like a great idea, but I've got too much on my plate right now."
"I can't take on the entire fundraising campaign, but I could organize one of the bake sales."

Then there are the big nos—the ones you have to say to a loved one or your overly demanding boss, where the personal or professional stakes are much higher. This is when you have to reach deep into your heart center, stand firm, and draw the line between you and what would be too much. This is why saying no takes practice. Finding this powerful center is like finding your balance in yoga. You'll find it; you'll wobble; you may even hit the mat. But keep at it, and it will grow easier to maintain over time.

The thing that most people get wrong about stress is that they wait until they are sick from it before getting serious about dealing with it. You can think of your personal energy like a bank account: You sleep well, you eat healthily, and you exercise regularly. Those are all deposits into your energy bank, and you think you're doing just fine. The problem is that most people think that it's the big life events that do us in, that create a catastrophic overdraft, but, in reality, it's the small stressors that nickel-and-dime us into ill health. Skipping your daily workout, eating junk food, and saying yes (or fine) when you really want to say no are small stressors chipping away at your reserves and that will ultimately leave you in the red. Translation? Chronic stress results in physical and emotional problems.

The better approach is to be consistent about checking in with yourself. Where are the stressors in your daily life? This is not the time to assign blame. Much like the process of responding to food cravings, it's important to slow down the process of responding to a stressor so that you can get a good look at it and decide how you want to respond. You may be surprised to learn that you have a choice in how you respond to stress. One of the most interesting things about my work as a counselor is the enormous range of reactions that people have in response to the same stressor. What will send one person over the edge is, for another person, no big deal. What that means is that there is not a strict rule to how to respond to stress, no such "If A happens, then I must B."

Further, just because you have responded to a particular stressor in the same way for years doesn't mean that you have to continue. If your repeated response hasn't resolved the stressor for you, it's okay to try another approach. In fact, if you're still struggling with the same stressor you had six months ago, you *need* to take a different approach. The most powerful question you can ask yourself when it comes to making lifestyle change is this: *What would happen if . . . ?*

As a woman with PCOS, avoiding stress is as important for you as is avoiding table sugar and sugary soda. Avoiding stress does not mean that you have to seal yourself in emotional bubble wrap. Occasional stress is a part of a full and healthy life. But handling stress with a positive, self-respectful mind-set is a powerful way to level up your life experiences and engagement in the world.

Of course, by handling stress with the intention of managing your PCOS, you will be taking powerful action to loosen the hormonal grip of cortisol, which will then allow your other lifestyle changes to be much more effective in reducing the symptoms of PCOS and improving your overall health.[2]

STRESS AND YOUR PHYSICAL HEALTH

According to the Holmes and Rahe stress scale, developed by psychiatrists over time to determine the correlation between life events and stress response,[3] the ten most stressful life events are the following, where 100 is the most stressful and 0 the least:

1. death of a spouse: 100
2. divorce: 73
3. marital separation: 65
4. imprisonment: 63
5. death of a close family member: 63
6. personal injury or illness: 53
7. marriage: 50
8. dismissal from work: 47
9. marital reconciliation: 45
10. retirement: 45

In order to measure a person's overall stress level using the Holmes-Rahe scale, the score is taken over a year-long period. When the total exceeds 300 points, there is high probability that some sort of illness will present within the next two years. If the score is between 150 and 299, the patient is at moderate risk of illness. Scores at 150 and under indicate a low probability of stress-related illness in the patient. It is worth noting that the top ten stressors are largely out of a person's control and that the Holmes-Rahe stressor list is by no means exhaustive. It simply serves to highlight the fact that we don't live in a bubble of peace and tranquility. Stressful situations can't always be avoided, so it's up to each person to manage inevitable stress with a combination of awareness, faith, support, and self-care.

Women with PCOS have additional life stressors that deserve to be acknowledged. Infertility, miscarriage, chronic pain, chronic illness, acne, absence of periods, and struggles with weight are all stress-inducing. Unfortunately, many women don't feel comfortable opening up about their struggles because they fear it will make them seem weak or ungrateful. They are worried that if they share the information, their concerns might be dismissed, making them feel ashamed—or at the very least frustrated.

PHYSICAL EFFECTS OF STRESS

The study by Holmes and Rahe confirmed what we have known for a long time: stress can lead to illness. There is no way to know how much stress is too much, nor can we accurately predict what sort of ailment will result from too much stress. But it is helpful for us to understand that there are similarities between a woman's physical response to PCOS and a person's physical response to stress. And it would not be too far a reach to consider that stress might make the stress response to dealing with those particular PCOS symptoms even worse.

Consider the following physiological responses to both PCOS and stress:

Headaches—Ranging from a sensation of tension around the temples to a migraine, headaches are one of the most common physical effects of stress. Typically, stress or tension headaches are felt around the forehead and the lower part of the back of the head. That said, tension headaches can trigger other types of headaches as well.

Digestive issues—Stress can affect every part of the digestion system. It can cause esophageal spasms, nausea, and either diarrhea or constipation. Medications like metformin can cause diarrhea, and stress has the potential to worsen the condition. Occasional stress, like an upcoming big game or important test, can cause occasional stomach upset that the body is capable of dealing with healthily. The situation becomes problematic when the stress is continuous, such as when a person is dealing with unresolved grief over infertility or with frustration about not being able to lose weight.

Blood pressure—Stress can cause a surge of hormones that constricts blood vessels and temporarily elevates blood pressure and can even cause chest pain. While there is no proof that chronic stress can raise blood pressure over the long term, elevated cortisol can damage arteries, which, over time, can lead to heart disease.

Chest pain—Stress usually leads to anxiety, which can trigger a panic attack. Panic attacks often include chest pain often mistaken for a heart attack. Always check with your doctor if you have any doubts about the cause of your chest pain.

Insomnia—Stress can rob you of deep, rejuvenating sleep and can even lead to chronic sleeplessness. Lack of sleep can raise cortisol, which makes insulin resistance worse. Many people deal with insomnia as a part of life, but sleep issues can be greatly improved with a better bedtime routine and adequate stress management. Medications for sleep are helpful for a few days but should be used in conjunction with changes in lifestyle. Managing insomnia will help you beat a common cause of fatigue. Being well rested helps control cravings and helps ensure you have enough energy for exercise and other self-care activities.[4]

Skin problems—Acne is one of the most common symptoms of PCOS. Stress causes acne, because it increases inflammation, which can in turn cause the pore to break and pus to form, creating what we commonly call a pimple. Stress also causes the adrenal gland to become overactive, which results in more testosterone. The additional testosterone leads to oilier skin and cystic acne.

Diabetes—Emotional stress causes higher glucose levels in the bloodstream. This is especially problematic for people with PCOS, as insulin resistance leads to more insulin being released. Eventually, the pancreas becomes fatigued and no longer produces sufficient amounts of insulin, resulting in type 2 diabetes.

Lowered immune system—Cortisol lowers the amount of lymphocytes in the blood. Lymphocytes are one of the building blocks of a healthy immune system. With fewer lymphocytes, the body is less able to fight off infection. In the most extreme cases, intense, long-term stress can cause so much inflammation that the immune system begins to attack the body, thinking that it is something foreign. This process is also known as *autoimmune disease*. And then the stress of having the autoimmune disease itself creates more stress, perpetuating the cycle further.[5]

"WHAT DOES IT MEAN TO MANAGE STRESS?"

Stress management isn't something you do once in a while or something you do in times of crisis. Stress management is continuous and goes hand-in-hand with resiliency.

Resiliency: Beating Stress before It Starts

We've talked about developing physical stamina through exercise, but a powerful bonus to regular physical activity is the development of emotional resilience. *Emotional resilience* is the ability to recover from stress. Stressful situations are a part of life, but they typically come and go. For many people, emotional resilience in the face of life's challenges can be the difference between stress remaining a short-term problem to cope with and a chronic issue.

Boundaries are essential to the development of emotional resilience. The key is finding the right balance: Boundaries that are too rigid can lead to problems with creating or maintaining healthy relationships. If you always say no, you miss out on opportunities for growth, exploration, and meaning in too many areas of your life. People will move on from trying to connect with you, or, if they are still around, they will struggle to understand the sort of help you need when you encounter difficulties.

However, boundaries that are too loose are equally problematic—and are more common for women. If you say yes when you know the answer should be no, then your boundary needs to be more boldly established. Loose boundaries make it especially difficult to manage stress. If you're saying yes to everything and everyone, then there is little time for self-care. In fact, the stress weighing you down might not be from the tasks themselves but from the frustration of saying yes to something you just don't want to do. Women can reduce stress in their lives just by strengthening those boundaries and speaking up for what they need and want. The challenge is making that consideration a part of your lifestyle rather than setting a hard-and-fast rule.

Following a wellness plan is fantastic and fun when everything is going well. Then? Life. Happens. You have to move or change jobs; someone gets sick—maybe there's a death in the family. And that wellness plan is imperiled.

Then What? How Do You Stay on Track?

Above all, understand that throughout your entire life you are in transition. What works for you right now might have to evolve over time. There is no rule book. The best approach to learning how to pivot and gracefully manage change is to treat yourself with love and respect. This is easier said than done, of course. But developing awareness through mindfulness ensures that you stay connected to stress levels, allowing yourself the opportunity to make adjustments before your health begins to suffer. You deserve to ease stress as much as anyone else.

After a life change or upon the introduction of a new stressor, depending on the situation, you may want to take a few days or more to reassess what your wellness plan resembles in light of your "new normal." If you are grieving, this is an especially important step for you to take, as grief includes a strong physical manifestation—almost like having the flu. The best thing you can do is nurture your body while it goes through the grieving process and then ease back into your exercise routine with a slow and mindful plan. No matter what, with every workout, you are creating emotional resilience. Have faith in the process. Though especially true for people grieving, this careful reassessment is valuable in every situation: Take a step back, and ask, *What can I learn here? How can I grow?* The answer may not be immediately apparent, but simply asking the question leaves the door open for insight later on.

You are stronger than you think—and braver too. How many times have you felt stressed and thought to yourself, *I can't handle this*, reaching for alcohol, cigarettes, or junk food? Any of these responses is a normal reaction to trying to escape stress. But you have to train your brain to sit with stress, and the benefits are worth the effort. One of the first things we were taught in counseling school was not to worry if you miss an issue in a session with a client because it will almost certainly come up again. The same is true for stress: If you escape from it, you lose the opportunity to do something about it, but if you trust your inner strength to sit with it for a while and keep an open mind about possible solutions, those solutions will come much more readily. And when you find a resolution, chances are that you won't experience that same stress again.

MEDITATION

Meditation is a practice that goes back thousands of years, but it is starting to find a way into today's mainstream culture. It has also started to receive praise from the medical community as an effective treatment for stress-related illness.

Johns Hopkins University reviewed nineteen thousand studies on meditation for health and then narrowed its focus onto forty-seven extremely well-designed studies. The researchers analyzed the data in those studies and found that a daily meditation practice reduces anxiety and stress and helps with pain management.[6] This means that for women with PCOS, meditation can help with stress management and anxiety reduction. This, in turn, leads to lower cortisol and improved insulin sensitivity. Meditation can improve sleep as well, leading to better control of your cravings and more energy overall. It can also help with reduction of inflammation, which is an underlying health concern, especially as it relates to autoimmune disease and cardiovascular disease.[7]

There are many different apps on the market for guided meditations; many of them are free outright (or at least offer free trials). If you think the idea of meditation sounds too New Agey, you will be pleasantly surprised to learn that meditation practice has grown to incorporate some methodologies that you might find a bit more relatable. Try several types of meditation practices before deciding it's not for you. I recommend looking into apps like Calm, Headspace, or Stop, Breathe, & Think, as a starting point.

As with any new habit, connect your new meditation practice with an activity that you already do consistently—like automatically taking five minutes to meditate after you brush your teeth in the morning—and try doing it at the same time every day. Meditation can be intense, so just do ten minutes a day at first and then gradually increase duration only as it feels comfortable. Let go of any concerns that you're not doing it correctly. Meditating when your mind is busy and stressed is like exercising when you are out of shape: you likely won't be able to come out of the first session feeling like a Buddhist monk any more than your first cardio session will turn you into an Olympic athlete. But there are benefits to be found in persistence, even in that first session, and the benefits continue to develop over time and with consistent practice.

If you find that you simply cannot meditate, don't despair! Exercises like walking and running are known as meditation in motion, offering the same benefits as meditation: improved energy, mental clarity, reduced anxiety, and more. You can also try simply deep breathing, in and out, for as long as it feels comfortable for you. Even one or two deep breaths during a stressful moment can help you calm down and release stressful feelings.

RELATIONSHIPS

If you have a few trusted and well-intentioned people whom you can call on when the going gets tough, then you are an incredibly lucky woman. From birth and throughout the rest of your time on Earth, life is all about growth. The quality of your relationships is the difference between constructively growing and merely coping. Whether you rely on connections with your family or on your family of choice, the bottom line is that they are in the ideal place to help you. They are close enough to know the whole story of you—good, bad, and ugly—but are removed enough to help you think through challenges with an objective perspective. Relationships are the collective consciousness. Done right, they will be the feedback you need to stay focused on living a full, balanced life.

IDENTIFYING STRESS

When we are talking about managing stress, we are really talking about taking our emotional pulse in every situation. Just because you can get through a situation doesn't mean that the stress has been managed. What are the stressful situations that keep coming up for you? Is it a routine doctor's visit? Chronic pain related to PCOS? Relationship problems due to infertility?

Stress management isn't about avoiding stress altogether, because that is nearly impossible. Instead, it's about deciding that you deserve to get the best possible result from every situation life throws at you. Once that decision is made, look for opportunities to put it into action. What are your familiar stressors? What keeps coming up for you that you tolerate? It's time to stop tolerating, because tolerating comes at the price of your health.

In any stress-reduction program, you have three possible courses of actions:

1. *Reduce the* frequency *of the stress*—This comes from setting better boundaries, valuing yourself more.
2. *Reduce the* intensity *of the stress*—Sit with the stress, taking steps to limit its effect, asking for help when you need it.
3. *Time management*—When it comes to setting better boundaries, learning how to best use your time and finite resources is beneficial. You learn to trust yourself and can get real about what you do and don't have time for. You can have the most beautiful exercise plan in the world, but if you don't value yourself and your time enough to do that exercise, then that plan won't be helpful. The reason it or any other act of self-care won't be helpful is because it's hard to be consistent when you're being pulled in many different directions at once, and consistent application is what makes or breaks any wellness plan. Then the whole situation is made worse when you feel guilty about taking time away for yourself. Guilt creates more stress. It's a vicious cycle.

Stress is ultimately what you make of it. While many stressful events aren't avoidable, there are plenty that are. The question is *Where do you put your energy?* Many people put it into identifying all of the ways that stress is hurting them. Another option is to acknowledge the stress, as if to say, *Okay, I see you there*, and mindfully move your attention away from it onto something else in your life that feels more manageable. Placing energy is like watering a plant: whatever receives your energy is what grows.

PERFECTION

Are you a perfectionist? Do you feel stressed out when things don't go according to plan? Is your life just not quite enough, despite your efforts?

Perfectionism is generally used to garner validation from someone. This feels necessary when you don't have a secure sense of self-worth. The need for perfection can cause anxiety, but the quest for perfection can create a long-term stress that is hard to shake.

Women with PCOS often struggle with a secure sense of self-worth. This is especially true when symptoms are more noticeable. The fact is that no external success will ever give you the secure sense of self-worth you are after. You are going to have to work that out as you go along. It's an ongoing process to maintain, but doing so allows you to spend more time in relaxed authenticity and less time feeling stressed because something didn't turn out the way you would have liked.

Letting go of the quest for perfection means that you have to embrace the chaos of life rather than resist it. Things come up without warning. Often the random events marring your quest for the ideal aren't malicious, aren't aimed at bringing you down personally, but they can feel that way when your hopes for perfection were resting on them.

Another way to disengage from the quest for perfection is to honor the principle of equifinality. This term, often used in management circles, refers to the many means to one end. Allowing for this—that there are myriad ways to achieve your goal—will save you a lot of stress. Keeping in mind the principle of equifinality helps you realize that you aren't the lynchpin to any given good outcome, that there are lots of solutions to the same problem, so it's okay and even helpful for you to set boundaries and say no when someone's trying to convince you that you just *have* to help. But even beyond boundary setting, the principle of equifinality helps us to just let go—letting go of our need to control the situation, manage every variable, and fight to make sure it turns out *just so*. And once we learn to let go, we've opened up a space for creativity and motivation to work their magic.

For example, you might have a plan detailing exactly how you want to change your diet and exercise program. You want it to be significant, and you want it implemented now. You have lists—mental or written, with bullet points!—and you have a timeline to go with that plan. Suddenly you realize that life is not getting with the program. If you were wed to your quest for perfection, you would likely get stuck in all-or-nothing thinking, and when your workouts became twenty minutes long instead of thirty, you would feel like a failure. With the principle of equifinality, however, you realize that your goal is to work out every day so that you consistently lose weight, and that means you might work out for ten minutes one day and thirty minutes the next but continually adhere to your goal. Implementing your wellness plan is a balancing act. And you reach your goal by ridding yourself of any stress that would lead you to burnout.

JOURNAL QUESTIONS

1. What stresses you? Make a list of your top ten stressors. Don't try to solve them. Simply list them so that you have a clear inventory. Put them in order, from most stressful to least. Next, circle the stressors you can change. Write out a plan to change at least one of those things this week.
2. What stressors do you choose to keep in your life? How would it feel if you simply weren't *allowed* to maintain them anymore?
3. What are at least five things that bring you joy?
4. When checking in with your body, are there some physical cues that stress is taking its toll?
5. What does "stress management" look like in your life? What, if anything, would you change?
6. What are at least five things you do when you get stressed? They can be positive or negative, but name the ones that you are *currently* doing. Chances are, you don't spend much time thinking about your stress-coping strategies. Considering them can get a little uncomfortable—because it's scary to imagine being left with no strategies at all.
7. What are the pros and cons to each strategy? Write them out specifically.

9

Mindfulness and Meditation

The Peaceful Healers

If you are depressed, you are living in the past.
If you are anxious, you are living in the future.
If you are at peace, you are living in the present.

—Lao-tzu

Mindfulness is the foundation of any good health strategy. While it is often presented in a way that feels overwhelming and unattainable, the truth is that being mindful simply means training your mind to notice thoughts and feelings in the present moment and allowing them to flow, resisting the urge to *do* something with them.

Mindfulness has its roots in Hinduism and Buddhism but has since evolved into a nonreligious practice. In 1979, it was introduced into Western culture by Jon Kabat-Zinn's mindfulness-based stress reduction (MBSR) program used to treat chronic illness. Later on, mindfulness-based cognitive therapy (MBCT) was developed to help people suffering from major depressive disorder.

No doubt, having PCOS is stressful; however, it is possible to reduce the degree of stress that is experienced.[1] The goal of mindfulness-based stress reduction is to disrupt any problematic functioning within the HPA axis, where the negative physical effects of stress originate.

No two people are the same. Everyone has their own strengths and challenges. As such, health plans should be adapted to the individual, not individuals to existing health plans. And mindfulness is how we make this happen.

> Mindfulness is the gentle effort to be continuously present with experience.
>
> —Bodhipaksa

HEALTH BENEFITS FOR WOMEN WITH PCOS

Mindfulness meditation reduces depression and anxiety. Mindfulness teaches us to notice when our mind is getting ahead of the game and to bring it back to the present moment. According to the original teachings of mindfulness, the present moment is the most natural state of the brain, so it is the healthiest and most comfortable.

In our culture, we often use drugs, alcohol, overeating, or other damaging strategies to cope with anxiety. The problem with those is that, though they might dull the discomfort of the anxiety for a brief period, they don't allow for personal growth or awareness in the moment. Some of the more powerful chemicals can dull the sense of being aware of potential problems, even if those concerns are valid. In the most extreme cases, relying on these inadequate coping mechanisms can develop into addiction to drugs or alcohol and engaging in life-threatening behavior like driving under the influence. Many addictions come with significant undesirable side effects. Mindfulness allows us to keep our wits about us so that we can make informed choices while at the same time allowing us to flow through the day. Mindfulness doesn't have to crash down on you in a mind-blowing moment of insight in order to be done well. Sometimes it's just a gentle awareness.

The best time to start a mindfulness practice is before you need it! Mindfulness is both a coping strategy and an act of self-care. It is a way to be more selective with your emotional reserves so that you spend that energy where and when you want to. This is how mindfulness creates the feeling of increased energy. It's not so much that you have more energy—although you *do* to some extent—but more that, once you begin a regular mindfulness practice, you will have more control of where you put your energy.

The paradox here is that you gain control by letting go of control. Instead of attending to each and every emotion you have—analyzing it, fighting it, or resolving it—what if you just let go? What if you just noticed your feelings without trying to make them go away? The fact is that the emotions that come up in you probably have every right to be there. It's perfectly okay to feel frustrated, sad, heartbroken, angry, or any of the other so-called negative feelings. Trying to act like you are positive, happy, optimistic, all the time, even when you aren't actually feeling any of those things, can leave you feeling like a fraud because you know your facade is not in alignment with reality. The goal is not to be happy all the time. It's exhausting to act like everything is fine when it really isn't. The feelings aren't wrong; the inauthenticity is the problem. The goal is to make space for your experience and use your energy judiciously to create a healthier life.

HOW TO DEVELOP YOUR MINDFULNESS PRACTICE

Mindfulness isn't a one-and-done exercise; it is a daily habit that needs to be maintained for greatest benefit. Fortunately, mindfulness can be done anywhere, any time. The difficulty is in breaking out of the habit of being reactionary to life and instead being present in the moment. Following are several different ways to develop mindfulness. I suggest you start with the practice that feels best for you and then expand into other options.

Simple Mindfulness Practice: Just Notice

Vietnamese Buddhist monk Thich Nhat Hanh recommends starting a mindfulness practice by simply noticing the world we live in.[2] For example, consider how often have you noticed the blue sky, and for a moment your awareness is focused solely on your gratitude for the blue sky. Nhat Hanh says we can expand this awareness to other moments in our life, and even the most mundane tasks can have a healing element to them when we become fully aware of them. Mindfulness meditation is more formal in that it is generally practiced at a specific time and with a specific intention. To make mindfulness part of your daily life, play with developing nonjudgmental awareness whenever you can, or at least whenever you feel stressed, depressed, or anxious.

Gratitude

Gratitude is a gift you give yourself that pays dividends in your health, well-being, and relationships. Typically, we reserve gratitude for the big things: a grand gesture from a friend, a medical miracle, healing from illness or injury. But the fact is that we have countless things to be grateful for every day. Wherever you direct your thoughts is what you will begin to see with consistency. This happens for several reasons, one being that our mind isn't as good at being multifocused as you might like to think. If you're focused on one thing, you lose perspective of all the other, potentially positive things in your life. For example, if you focus your thoughts on your acne, your mind will be trained to make your acne relevant in every area of your life. Life with PCOS can be challenging enough as it is, but if you give it all of your energy, you miss out on how strong you are or the amazing contributions you bring to your work.

To enjoy the healing effects of gratitude, it is not enough to simply say that you are grateful when you are prompted to think about it. Gratitude is a perspective that must become a well-established mind-set. Fortunately, with improved sleep, strengthened relationships, and increased happiness, the positive effects of a gratitude habit make it an enjoyable practice to maintain.[3]

Finding opportunities to practice gratitude isn't difficult, as there are an infinite number of things to be grateful for. You can be grateful for your family, but get specific. The only difficult part of the practice is in looking past any anger or resentment to acknowledge the good things in your life. This is easier said than done, but it is possible. Focusing on the good doesn't make the bad less valid; it simply allows your full story to develop.

One of the most uplifting and self-reinforcing ways to establish a gratitude practice is to keep a gratitude journal. To start, decide whether you want to devote yourself to the practice early in the morning or just before bedtime. Doing it first thing in the morning sets the tone for your day. Doing it at night can help you ease the stress of the day and help you more peacefully transition to sleep.

Next, write down three things you are grateful for.

Now, repeat this practice at the same time, every day. Set an alert on your phone to remind you until it is a confirmed habit.

TIP: When you are adding a new habit to your life, try to attach it to another habit that is already established. For example, if you choose to keep a gratitude journal in the morning, you might decide to do it while you enjoy your morning coffee. Linking the two activities reduces the gap between intention and action.

Meditation

Meditation is a type of mindfulness. A practice going back thousands of years, today meditation is increasingly recognized in the mainstream as an effective treatment for stress and anxiety.

Most people who don't like the idea of meditation are at odds with its perceived religious ties—and perhaps with mindfulness in general. But what they may not realize is that meditation has been used worldwide in secular settings to improve health, manage stress, and improve performance. Yes, it certainly can be used to deepen your spiritual experience if you choose. But it is not necessarily tied to any one religion, and it does not have to be at all. Simply put, meditation is a way to stay present in your mind, your body, and your life. It can help sharpen your focus, relax your nervous system, and deepen your experience of the "now."

Meditation can be effectively practiced in a variety of ways as long as you're setting aside time to make yourself feel good. Repetitive, more solitary exercises like running, walking, or swimming can allow the mind to reach a meditative state. Listening to music with meditative intention can be effective.

The results of one highly regarded meta-study analyzing the effects of meditation practice confirmed that for people who had mild to moderate feelings of anxiety and depression, mindfulness meditation was as effective as medication and without any side effects.[4]

Mindfulness-based stress reduction is an eight-week in-person program that includes one two-hour class per week, along with one six-hour retreat. Participants are expected to meditate for forty-five minutes a day. In addition, they are taught simple yoga moves as well as the mindfulness technique known as body scanning. Usually done with in-person training, MBSR, as it is known, is increasingly practiced with the help of online resources. Many studies have demonstrated a connection between MBSR and stress reduction. Close to 80 percent of medical schools offer some sort of mindfulness training, and it has been the subject of numerous research studies. On the whole, these studies indicate that MBSR in particular is effective in managing even extreme stress reactions, like the effects of post-traumatic stress disorder and chronic pain, and can even reduce the inflammation that leads to heart disease.

Mindfulness-based cognitive therapy—or MBCT—is similar to MBSR in terms of format and approach. The only difference is that MBCT was designed to help people with depression, so the focus of that eight-week series goes straight to identifying low mood and developing strategies to change that. Studies indicate that mindfulness meditation can improve outcomes in chronic pain, depression, anxiety, and drug addiction. MBSR also lowers the inflammatory response. Inflammation is an insidious player in PCOS and in many chronic illnesses. Researchers believe this is primarily due to stress hormones like cortisol.

Addiction is a significant roadblock to both mental and physical health. Whether the addiction is with food, alcohol, drugs, something else altogether, or any combination thereof, mindfulness meditation can help. First, it can help you become more comfortable with the present moment, which is usually what people are trying to escape when they take their drug of choice. Mindfulness meditation also helps reduce impulsivity and improve self-control, which can go far in preventing relapse. It also helps improve control of cravings, as it teaches you to be aware of the cravings in a very real way rather than simply reacting to them.

Pain control is also enhanced by mindfulness meditation, as it can help distract from the pain as well as the experience of the pain itself. While various distraction techniques have long been employed to manage pain, recent studies have shown that practitioners of mindfulness meditation learn to manage their pain even more efficiently and effectively.[5] And this includes managing psychological pain: the benefits of mindfulness for people suffering from anxiety and depression include reduced self-criticism, reduced rumination about the past, and reduced worrying about the future.

Body Scanning

Strengthening the body-mind connection is enormously helpful in maintaining motivation for a healthy lifestyle change. Body scanning isn't about creating new information; it is about noticing and interpreting the information that has been there all along so that you can make informed decisions about what your body and mind need.

Getting this information allows you to make adjustments to emotional reactions. Anger, overwhelm, and fear can all interfere with your wellness efforts, so their effective clearing can be useful. The problem is that most women are completely out of touch with their bodies. This makes consistency in self-care difficult to maintain. Lack of connection to your body means that you get further and further off track from healthy self-care practices before noticing there is a problem. Imagine touching a hot stove, but the neural connection is poor, so the pain message moves more slowly, resulting in a delay and greater injury before you know to move your hand away from the heat. Being in tune with what our body is experiencing and feeling helps us course correct more quickly at the earliest onset of a problem.

> The body says what words cannot.
>
> —Martha Graham

Body scans facilitate the development of a more efficient early-warning system for stress, anxiety, depression, and more. Over time and with practice, you learn to associate physical sensations with the calibration of your well-being.

If you struggle with binge eating, body scanning can help you identify stressors that typically trigger a binge. Understanding this connection in advance gives you the opportunity to take action ahead of time and outright remove the stressor if necessary, but it also gives you the opportunity to dismiss the stressor from your thoughts entirely if it becomes a ruminating thought or other unpleasant feeling.

What would happen if you didn't grin and bear it? Stoicism merely expands the gap between mind and body and ends up being detrimental to public health. And it's even worse for women with PCOS who struggle most with weight gain and other symptoms; having a stiff upper lip cures nothing. Instead, increasing awareness of the body can make all the rest of the habits you've incorporated into your wellness plan even more effective and lasting.

And the best part? All the technique requires of you is that you *notice*.

In body scanning, participants are invited to give attention to every part of their bodies, from their toes to the top of their heads. Body scanning is helpful for people with food issues and obesity, because sufferers of these disorders tend to be out of touch with their bodies. And both dysfunctional relationships with food and obesity are common among women with PCOS. While body scanning may seem simple, its results can be profound. How often do you mindlessly ignore, or worse, criticize your body?

Mindfulness has at its core the following ideas:

Not being judgmental—Have you ever been close to someone who would take every opportunity to criticize you? Criticism destroys relationships. And so, too, is constantly judging yourself destructive. Habitually judging your every thought can keep you on edge, never able to truly accept yourself. Practicing being nonjudgmental is a powerful step toward relaxing into self-acceptance.

Not striving—This pillar of mindfulness is the reminder that the only thing we have to give energy to is what is here right now. Resisting the urge to be, do, and have takes discipline but is worth the effort.

Acceptance—Mindfulness teaches us that in order to make any changes we must first go all-in accepting ourselves for who we are right now.[6] Women with PCOS may find this difficult to accept. Who wants to do all that life-transformation work for someone she doesn't even really like? But without acceptance, positive, healthy changes are impossible. Remember, it is perfectly healthy to love yourself and still want better for yourself. As Maya Angelou said, "When you know better, you do better." As you learn healthier ways of being from this book, it is perfectly okay to love yourself where you are now and still apply the principles for change.

Letting go—Perhaps the hardest skill in any mindfulness program is finding the balance in how you respond to your thoughts. On the one hand, you don't want to go looking for your thoughts or striving for the "right" ones. Nor is rejecting passing thoughts productive, because typically attempting to dispel them keeps them rebounding right back, obsessively, entirely defeating the purpose. The goal, rather, is a curious, gentle awareness and a mindful release of those thoughts.

Cultivating the beginner's mind—Your body isn't a machine, so it stands to reason that your mind isn't one, either. While it may feel like you should build from one skill or one insight to the next in a step-by-step manner, the best approach to cultivating mindfulness is to stay open to new developments, ask questions, and treat each attempt with the same curiosity and energy you would if you were first trying it.

Resist the urge to expect the development of mindfulness excellence, as it will make results harder to come by.

Patience—Results might not happen overnight. Being patient in your mindfulness will allow for consistency. This is the foundation of any mindfulness practice and the one that most people struggle with.

Trust—If you're lucky, you have that one person in your life to whom you can say anything, the one you know who won't judge you or reject you. Often people long for this connection without realizing that this is a gift they can give themselves. Mindfulness can free you to trust yourself enough to notice all of your thoughts and feelings without having to brace yourself for harsh inner criticism.

Noncentering—Also known as *decentering*, this is one of the pillars of mindfulness that gives the most emotional benefit. It is the belief that thoughts and feelings can come and go without being internalized or causing you to label yourself. If you struggle with anxiety or depression, this practice can be incredibly therapeutic. For example, when you find yourself focusing on a particular worry, noncentering asks you to identify the worry as just that—a worry, nothing more. Once you are able to notice your thoughts and truly see them for what they are—a thought, neither a reality nor a prediction—it's easier to dismantle the persistent worry, recognize that it has no value, and release it. Practicing this strategy can reverse, or at least effectively manage, generalized anxiety.

WHEN YOU ~~CAN'T~~ *DON'T* MEDITATE

If you hate meditating or feel like you can't meditate, then you're not alone. Many people struggle with preconceived notions of what it means to meditate—like achieving complete inner calm or blithely chanting inexplicable mantras—and decide that it's not a good fit. But just as it is with exercise, the benefits of meditation are not enough to make you like it and keep doing it; you have to find what you like and ease into it. There are many types of meditation, many of which don't involve sitting in the lotus position for an hour a day while you listen to New Age music. For many of us, that would feel inauthentic or even fraudulent.

Women are accustomed to wearing multiple hats. Shifting among those responsibilities throughout the day can create a sense of pressure, urgency, and, ultimately, anxiety. Meditation, and especially mindfulness meditation, stands in direct yet gentle contrast to that busy mind and life-style and can alleviate the anxiety that goes with it.

But meditating doesn't have to be daunting. Unfortunately, meditation has gotten a reputation for being intense and time consuming. The reality is that, just as in exercise, you can get tremendous benefit from dialing back the intensity of your meditation practice so that it's less intimidating and more consistent. Many downloadable apps provide guided meditations that can be done in as few as six minutes. For some people, starting slow is the way to go. If you can build your practice, great; if you can't, don't worry about it—meditation is not meant to be judgmental. Whatever you can fit in, whatever feels best for you in your daily life, is what you should do. If you can find a part of your day to sit with your thoughts and let your mind focus on the breath, the body, and the present, you may find the benefits reach beyond just your immediate health concerns. You may find greater focus. Greater patience. Greater love for your life and everything in it. And if you don't, that's fine, too.

Here are some tips to making meditation a consistent part of your healthy lifestyle:

> *Set aside your prejudgments*—Not all meditation practices are created equal. If you don't like one, try another. Mindfulness meditation has been documented to have practical applications in improving outcomes for women with chronic stress, anxiety, and depression, but it is not the only approach. Just like there are many ways to exercise, there are many ways to meditate; there is no right or wrong. It is simply a matter of finding what works for you.
>
> *You have enough time to meditate*—If you worry that you are too busy to incorporate a new meditation practice into your chaotic life, keep in mind that a commitment to a ten-minute meditation practice can help you become more emotionally grounded, putting your energy where it serves you best and not into suffering with anxiety, depression, and critical self-talk. I recommend starting with a consistent practice of guided meditation for ten minutes every morning. This can set the tone for the healthy lifestyle choices you make throughout the rest of your day.
>
> *Racing thoughts needn't derail your meditation practice*—If you struggle with a busy mind while you meditate, it can be an anxiety-provoking challenge to sit quietly with them. It can feel too vulnerable. The point of meditation is not to work through your emotional

challenges; rather, the point is to train your brain to work in a more balanced and productive way. Mindfulness meditation teaches us to be a nonjudgmental observer of those thoughts, which can be a relief.

Find the meditational practice that best works for you and your needs— For example, if you suffered trauma as a child, then any meditation that asks you to imagine yourself as a child might be a trigger and ultimately unhelpful. And while mindfulness meditation has been shown to be useful for people who suffer from post-traumatic stress disorder, I recommend that if you suffer from PTSD or any other severe mental-health challenge, you should work with a qualified professional to find the meditation practice that meets you where you are. For example, your hidden coping strategies for PTSD might be more effective than you think, and removing them suddenly could cause some serious upset.

A restless body can learn to be still—If your body is restless in meditation, there could be a few things going on: First, you might have a lot of nervous energy that is longing to be channeled efficiently. Daily exercise can help this issue. A second possible cause for your restlessness could simply be that you aren't in the right position; sitting in a posture that's unfamiliar or uncomfortable makes it hard to settle into meditation. And while many meditation practitioners make specific recommendations for how you should sit, the reality is that you should sit in whatever way feels right for you. If that means sitting up in a chair, assuming the lotus position, or lying flat on the floor, it's fine—so long as your positioning keeps you as comfortable and natural as possible.

There's no one right way to meditate—While the specifics vary from person to person, many people have a concern with meditation that they aren't doing it correctly. This is based in self-criticism and pre-judgment. There is no right or wrong way to meditate, because each person is on her own path. Even guided meditations are merely suggestions. There is no pinnacle of meditational achievement, and meditation is most definitely not a competition. It's a lifelong practice, just like a healthy diet and exercise. There will be easier days and harder days. The point is to accept it without judgment. However your mind is wandering, just being mindful of it is healing in and of itself.

Apply meditation to your life—Formal mindful meditation practice is just the beginning. Much like learning about a healthy lifestyle, the beauty of mindful meditation happens when it's applied to the many decisions you make throughout your day. Attention can only be maintained for about three or four seconds. That's it! You can do anything for a few seconds at a time. The truth is that your attention is supposed to wander off. It's completely normal. Mindfulness can be as simple and fast as taking a moment out of your day to be aware of what you're thinking, doing, smelling, and feeling. Mindfulness is the combined effect of multiple tiny decisions to be present that in turn creates progressive development and a deeper, more secure sense of calm.

JOURNAL QUESTIONS

1. Why do you want to be more present with your family and friends? What's hard about that?
2. What are the behaviors that distract you the most? (For example, checking social media and e-mail, watching TV, etc.)
3. How do you show it when you're present and actively listening to others?
4. What does your inner critic tend to say? Write her a letter explaining how you *feel* about her opinion. Try to explain how your life will improve without additional criticism.

10

Dealing with Symptoms of PCOS

PCOS brings with it obvious physical manifestations. While these physical symptoms are not necessarily a health concern, their emotional impact can be devastating and is impossible to ignore. In this chapter, some
of the more common symptoms of PCOS are introduced along with typical
interventions. It's important to talk with your health-care team, do your research, and choose the interventions and treatments that are right for you.

ACNE

Common acne, known as *acne vulgaris*, is caused by bacteria on the top
layers of the skin. When a pore gets clogged with dirt and bacteria, a
whitehead can form. This type of acne responds well to topical treatments
such as benzoyl peroxide or salicylic acid, both found in over-the-counter
treatments. Common acne also responds well to changes in diet, including
reducing or eliminating dairy and fried foods. However, for women with
PCOS, these interventions are not enough.

Cystic acne is a common symptom of PCOS and much more severe and
serious than common acne. It's also one of the most upsetting symptoms
of PCOS, as it can be very noticeable when it forms on the jawline, chest,
and back. Cystic acne is different from more common forms of acne in that
it forms larger and deeper lesions. They are painful, take a long time to
heal, and can leave scars. Studies of quality of life for women with PCOS

indicate that acne has a tremendous impact, especially when it comes to self-esteem, so it is worth the investment to address it.[1]

Women with cystic acne often fare better with the help of medical intervention. The reason for this is that this type of acne is often more than a minor bacterial infection. For women with PCOS, cystic acne is caused by increased testosterone in the skin. The increased testosterone increases oil production within the sebaceous glands, but rather than sitting on the surface of the skin, the oil clogs pores from within, meaning that no matter what skin products you use, no matter how diligent your routine, the acne will persist.

Some women have seen a slight improvement in their cystic acne when they cut out dairy, which contains lactose, a sugar. The suggestion is that less dairy results in less sugar in the bloodstream, less sugar results in less testosterone, and less testosterone results in less oil production, which creates less acne.

Patience Is a Virtue

There are several medical options to treating cystic acne—each with its own risks and benefits, so don't take any medication without first consulting your OBGYN or dermatologist. Because the treatments for PCOS-related acne are hormonally related, it's important to take the medication exactly as directed and avoid missing doses. If you choose to take medication for your cystic acne, keep in mind that it can take weeks, even months, to see positive results. In fact, your acne is likely to get worse before it gets better. I recommend waiting at least three months before making a judgment about the effectiveness of your medication. The reason for this is because cystic acne is not a superficial issue but part of a larger cycle of events; it takes time for medications to adjust hormone levels, and once those hormone levels are adjusted, it takes more time still for pores to be unclogged of overproduced oil and for any bacterial infections under the skin to clear up before you will see discernable results.

Spironolactone is one common treatment for PCOS-related acne. A diuretic, it was originally used as a treatment for heart disease and high blood pressure. Doctors and researchers were surprised to learn that it is incredibly effective in reducing androgens like testosterone.[2] It is important to drink enough water to avoid dehydration while taking spironolactone because of its diuretic properties. Also, take care not to eat too many bananas or other potassium-rich foods while on this medication, as these can cause unsafe levels of potassium in the body. Talk to your doctor or dietician to establish safe levels of consumption if these types of foods are a significant part of your diet. It may take several months to see the full effectiveness of spironolactone, but for many women, the result is clear skin and less unwanted hair growth. *This medication should not be taken by women who are trying to become pregnant, as it has been known to cause birth defects.*[3]

Birth control pills are commonly used to help women lower androgen levels. By managing their hormones, many women are able to reduce acne, excess hair growth, insulin resistance, and cystic ovaries. In addition, birth control pills can help regulate menstrual cycles. If you are over the age of thirty-five, are a smoker, or have a history of cardiovascular issues, be sure to talk to your doctor about the risks and benefits of taking a birth control pill.

Finding the Right Doctor

Cystic acne is one of the simplest of the PCOS-related symptoms to treat. For most women, it's not necessary to go to a dermatologist to treat it, since your doctor or endocrinologist can likely prescribe something that will help with the hormonal imbalance typically causing the cystic acne. That said, if your acne is severe or combined with other skin problems, then talking to a dermatologist can be helpful. Be sure to take notes from each doctor visit about what intervention was decided upon and share all medical interventions among your doctors so that everyone is on the same page. Because time is of the essence in a doctor's visit, it can be helpful to bring along a printed list of doctors treating you and medications you are taking.

Tips on Managing Acne

Cystic acne is a very common symptom of PCOS and also one of the most upsetting. Cystic acne is different from the typical "teenage" acne in that it is a deeper, larger lesion—a cyst—and it does not respond well to over-the-counter medications. Many women struggle with cystic acne for years before asking their doctor for help. If you have cystic acne, there are a few things to keep in mind:

> *Don't pick at your acne*—Opening a cyst can introduce more infection into the broken skin. Pushing on a cyst can spread infection to other

areas under the skin. Broken skin is much harder to conceal with makeup (if you choose to use it) and can lead to scarring.

Don't hate your skin—While it's understandable, it's not helpful. Harsh chemicals and aggressive treatment usually make the problem worse.

Be careful about the products you use on your face—If you choose to cover your acne with makeup, make sure that the makeup you choose won't clog pores. Check out video tutorials about makeup techniques to cover acne. Not only are they helpful, but it's also comforting to remember that you are not alone with this challenge.

Avoid exposing your skin to hot water—Wash your face with lukewarm water. Hot water strips all the oil off of your face and stimulates your oil glands to overproduce.

Keep your doctor in the loop about any home remedies you're using—While certain home remedies can help with inflammation and reduce the size and pain of cysts, they are rarely effective enough to disrupt a powerful hormonal cycle. Be sure to mention to your doctor any home treatments you're using. Granted, they are seeing everything from a medical perspective and likely have very little knowledge of natural solutions; however, they can tell whether something is likely to be harmful. Otherwise, if it doesn't hurt and it might help, then your home remedy is probably okay.

What you eat affects your skin—Women vary on their sensitivity, but your diet can definitely have a significant effect on your skin. It's often a good idea to avoid dairy products, sugars, and simple carbohydrates—basically, any food that causes inflammation. I don't recommend going on extreme diets, however, because they're not sustainable.

EXCESS HAIR (HIRSUTISM)

Hirsutism is excess hair growth in areas where one would typically see hair growth in only men, affecting between 5 and 10 percent of women of reproductive age.[4] PCOS is the most common cause of hirsutism, making up 70 percent of all cases. Excess hair is a symptom of higher testosterone in the system. While there is no medical need to manage the hirsutism itself, it usually causes significant emotional pain and can lower a woman's assessment of her quality of life. As a result, some sort of intervention is generally regarded as helpful. The best approach is a combination of medication, cosmetic procedures, and, in some cases, emotional support.

Medication

The effectiveness of medical treatments for excess hair growth varies from woman to woman. The most common medical intervention is the use of spironolactone. Some birth control pills can be helpful in treating mild hirsutism and are considered a first line of treatment. Metformin is not associated with an improvement in hirsutism.

Cosmetic Procedures

Cosmetic procedures like electrolysis and laser hair removal must be done by trained professionals. Significant burns and infection can occur if the procedures are done improperly. Not all states are regulated. If you can't travel to a state that is regulated, ask to see credentials that the person performing the procedure is a certified medical electrologist, a certified clinical electrologist, or a certified professional electrologist. Ask to have a fifteen-minute spot test of any procedure you are considering. If there is any damage to your skin after the treatment or you don't like the effectiveness of the hair removal, then you know it's time to try either another approach or a different practitioner.

If you would prefer at-home treatments for laser hair removal or electrolysis, Amazon or a targeted Google search is useful for comparing product prices, reading reviews of their efficacy, and exploring other options. Be sure to do your research on any hair-removal tools and machines, as they vary in quality and effectiveness.

Electrolysis

Electrolysis is a slower, very precise procedure and so generally ideal for small areas. The benefit of electrolysis is that it is the only FDA-approved approach for *permanent* hair removal. Galvanic electrolysis is the oldest method and involves sending a small electric current into the hair follicle. Thermolysis is a type of electrolysis that uses radio waves to create heat that damages the hair follicle; it is faster than galvanic electrolysis and can be used on all skin and hair colors. There is also a combination of these two approaches, known as the Blend, which many people feel gets the best results.

Laser Hair Removal

Laser hair removal is an option for larger areas. The laser is a flash of light that feels like being popped with a hot rubber band. It damages anything that is darker, so this option is best for women with dark hair on light skin. It is not an option for women with darker skin or lighter-colored hair. It may require several treatments for lasting effect but is not considered a permanent option.

Waxing, Plucking, and Shaving

While waxing and plucking isn't permanent and can cause significant irritation, it does slow the growth of stubble. To avoid infection, choose a quality salon with a licensed esthetician.

Shaving is a lower-cost, at-home remedy but must be done every day for cosmetic benefit. It can cause skin irritation, and many women say that it makes their acne worse.

ANDROGENIC ALOPECIA (HAIR LOSS)

Androgenic alopecia is thinning of hair or baldness that affects approximately 22 percent of women suffering from PCOS.[5] It is caused by excess testosterone in the body that converts to dihydrotestosterone (DHT), a hormone that has a tendency to move toward the scalp, clogging hair follicles, causing hair to fall out, and inhibiting regrowth. It usually appears as a receding hairline and a wider part on the top of the head.

Medications

Finasteride is the only oral medication FDA-approved for treatment of androgenic alopecia. It works by reducing the DHT in the system. Spironolactone is also often used with a possible benefit, since it also reduces testosterone in the system. It's important to know that positive results aren't guaranteed with medication, and it is not a permanent solution.

Topical Treatments

Minoxidil (trademarked as Rogaine) is an over-the-counter topical treatment that can temporarily slow hair loss and even help with hair regrowth in some cases. It is not a permanent solution, as the hair regrowth is dependent on continued use.

Lifestyle strategies for androgenic alopecia are similar to treatments for most other symptoms of PCOS. Reducing testosterone in the system along with lifestyle strategies like consistent exercise, appropriate diet, and adequate sleep can stop and even reverse hair loss.

ACANTHOSIS NIGRICANS (AN)

Acanthosis nigricans is a common condition where patches of the skin become darker and thicker, taking on what is often described as a velvety or dirty appearance. It is typically seen around the neck, armpits, or thighs but can also appear on the face. AN is typically not a medical issue; however, the cosmetic concern can cause emotional pain and affect quality of life. AN is a symptom of insulin resistance. While laser therapy and topical treatments are helpful in some cases, reducing the cause—insulin resistance—is the primary treatment of choice. For this purpose, medications like metformin can be helpful, along with weight loss as a result of lifestyle changes.

INFERTILITY

Very often women don't realize that they have PCOS until they seek out help for infertility. PCOS is the leading cause of anovulatory infertility—that is, infertility due to lack of ovulation.[6] Normally, women ovulate once a month. Unlike men, who make new sperm all the time, women are born with all of the eggs they will ever have, already in their ovaries. Ovaries are normally about the size of a walnut. Eggs, which are smaller than a grain of sand, are held in a blister-like follicle on the ovary. Gonadotropins are hormones released by the anterior pituitary gland. The main gonadotropins are follicle-stimulating hormone (FSH) and luteinizing hormone (LH). FSH stimulates the follicle to grow; after about two weeks, the follicle is about the size of a grape. After the follicle has grown to full size, ovulation is triggered by a surge in LH—the hormone detected in home-ovulation test kits.[7] Ovulation occurs when the follicle ruptures and the egg is released to be carried off through the fallopian tube for possible fertilization by sperm.

For women with PCOS, ovulation doesn't usually go this smoothly. Many women with PCOS don't have a regular period, which is part of the menstrual cycle. Along with higher androgens, women with PCOS have lower FSH and higher LH. Low FSH means the follicles don't reach maturity. High LH results in a lack of the surge in hormone that triggers the release of the egg.[8] This is what leaves the ovaries covered in cysts. Any follicle larger than two centimeters is considered a cyst; however, cysts can be as large as an orange. Cysts will either rupture or simply be absorbed by the body.[9]

LH is controlled by the HPA axis. High LH leads to low FSH, which causes increased testosterone to be released from the ovaries. It is because of this hormone imbalance that women with PCOS don't have a regular period.

While overweight women and extremely underweight women are less likely to ovulate, the good news is that diet and lifestyle changes can make a difference. For women who are overweight, weight loss of 5–10 percent can often restore ovulation. This is one area where medications and lifestyle strategies can work together beautifully. The goal is to use both approaches so that one enhances the effect of the other.

Women with PCOS also have a harder time maintaining pregnancy due to low progesterone. If you've been diagnosed with PCOS, it can be helpful to talk to your doctor when you are ready to start trying to get pregnant, as progesterone supplementation can help support pregnancy in the early stages.

Whether you have PCOS or not, miscarriages sometimes happen—and much more often than anyone talks about. If you have had a miscarriage, please know that you are not alone and that support and resources are available.

Medications can very often restore fertility by stimulating ovulation. Clomid (generically, clomiphene) is a medication that blocks estrogen receptors in the brain and raises FSH and LH, which helps to develop an egg follicle and then release the egg for possible fertilization. The main side effect is increased mood swings and abdominal cramping, but others exist, so it is important to talk with your doctor about whether this medication is right for you. Femara (generically, letrozole) is another medication that raises FSH so that the follicle can develop; this drug is a good option if the patient doesn't tolerate Clomid well. If Clomid and Femara are unsuccessful, women can opt for injectable gonadotropins, LH and FSH. This can be a little more expensive, and giving yourself a shot can be difficult; however, the success rate for inducing ovulation is 90 percent, assuming there are no other causes of infertility. Pregnancy rates after injection are also better than when Clomid was used.

Regardless of the medical course you follow, you must be monitored regularly by a doctor while taking the medications. Some drugs can result in too many mature follicles being released, and high-order multiples can be conceived. An infertility doctor can walk you through the best options and will monitor you closely to see what works best.

One benefit to PCOS is that your fertility *improves* with age as testosterone naturally drops.[10] Women with PCOS have an additional two years of fertility compared to women who don't have PCOS.

JOURNAL QUESTIONS

1. In terms of the physical symptoms of PCOS, what is your biggest concern?
2. How will an improved lifestyle help you with these symptoms?
3. If you're considering cosmetic treatment, how do think your life will improve? Are there any drawbacks to treatment?

11

❖ ❖

Creating Your Wellness
Dream Team

Imagine that your body is a successful company with many divisions and you its CEO. Many departments come together to achieve your goal: total wellness. Your job isn't to know and do everything. Instead, your goal is to embrace the vision and organize team efforts to achieve it. Knowing what teams you need and when you need them is crucial to your success. To have a successful team, your team doesn't need to be motivated by you; they already have their own motivation. You only have to remove any roadblocks that might hinder their progress. As the company of You grows and changes, you may need to add, take away, or change the departments. You know what being healthy means to you. It's time to make that vision a reality with the confidence and precision of a CEO.

This chapter is all about selecting your dream team of health-care providers and figuring out how to nurture those relationships for the best possible experience and outcome. You might not need all of these professionals at once, but it's important to know how to partner with them effectively when you do. If you do have more than one type of provider, then you are the organizer who will help them connect with accuracy and efficiency. Having the right team can improve your health care and lower your stress.

DOCTORS

The average amount of time that a doctor spends with a patient is between thirteen and sixteen minutes. It's actually amazing how much care a doctor provides while they are in the room with you.[1] Granted, there is variation, but considering this average, there is a lot that can be communicated if you manage your time properly.

Most women with PCOS are working with their OBGYN. This is probably because before an official PCOS diagnosis is made, the woman seeks medical help in the absence of regular periods or when she has trouble conceiving. Working with your OBGYN is the perfect place to start and may be all the help you need. But there are other health-care options that may enhance your experience and help you find better results. Endocrinologists specialize in conditions and diseases caused by hormones. If your PCOS is not improving with the standard treatments, or if you have other conditions that complicate matters, then partnering with an endocrinologist can be extremely helpful.

Doctors will generally take the lead in an office visit because most patients come in to be treated, not to be a participant in the process. Stepping into the role of an active participant in the treatment process is not only efficient but also incredibly empowering. Your doctor has all of the medical knowledge, but there is only so much that can be done if she doesn't get any feedback from you.

If you don't like your doctor, it's okay to change. That said, if every doctor in town seems to have the same problem, it may be time to consider whether your expectations or insecurities might be affecting your care. Are you shooting the messenger? PCOS and its related symptoms can cause significant stress and upset. It's normal to want the source of your stress to go away as soon as possible. If having PCOS is making you feel vulnerable and angry, it's helpful to acknowledge this situation and try to work with your doctor with an open mind. Are you feeling heard? Is there anything else you'd like to share at the appointment?

Whether your doctor has the personality or bedside manner you would prefer matters less than her understanding of the many nuances of PCOS and its treatment. We are programmed to feel at ease with people who match our communication style and emotional states. When you have PCOS, the stakes feel high and you naturally come to the appointment with feelings of nervousness and even anger. Your doctor likely won't share that energy, and that's a good thing, even if it feels a bit off. You want a doctor who will give you accurate and complete information and diligently craft a medical solution that is right for you. Here's the hard truth: When it comes to diagnosing PCOS, your doctor's job is fairly simple. The medical interventions that follow a diagnosis will vary, but the responsibility is on you to follow through with her recommendations and make the lifestyle changes necessary. All the medication in the world can't undo the impact of an unhealthy lifestyle. Resist the urge to go from doctor to doctor until you get a quick fix. There isn't one.

The following details the different types of doctors you might select to be a part of your dream team, as well as suggestions for clearing any roadblocks to care and making the most of the partnership.

In order to get the best care from your doctor, you should:

Make sure that each doctor is aware of the other one—Have each doctor's name and number available to share. This is helpful if your doctor has a question about lab results or treatment plans.

List all of your medications, carefully noting the dosage—Many people bring their medications with them, which is perfectly fine too. This is especially important if you are on multiple medications. Medications can interact with one another with dangerous results. The same is true for supplements. Remember, just because something is "all-natural" doesn't mean it's necessarily safe when used in combination with other medications. Include them on the list, and let your doctor decide what is relevant. There are also apps that can keep all this information organized for you.

Be honest—If you have no intention of taking a medication that was prescribed, it's best to be honest about it so that you don't waste time. It is possible that your resistance is coming from a place of not having enough information. Very often this problem can be cleared up with a few more questions.

Write down your questions before your visit—Sometimes it's hard to remember them all when you're in the moment.

Write down the answers to your questions and any new information—A doctor's visit brings a certain degree of stress that can make remembering details difficult.

Take any Internet-based information with a grain of salt—The Internet is a fantastic place to gather information, but it's not always accurate. All it takes is one official-looking article written by someone trying to sell the newest supplement for you to start doubting your treatment plan. If you have a question about the safety or effectiveness of your doctor's approach, by all means ask, and be sure to give your doctor's response a fair hearing.

Respect your doctor's time—Arrive at your appointment fifteen minutes early.

Keep an open mind—You may feel that your doctor isn't as intense about your case as you think she should be. While your PCOS is a unique life event for you, your doctor has likely seen similar cases several times that day already. The solution lies in effort and understanding from both sides.

NURSES

Be nice to the nurses. Seriously. Nurses are not there simply to be an assistant. Nurses bring their own strengths and expertise to your care. They are your bonus provider and can be powerful allies with the knowledge to help bridge the gap between being assigned a treatment and making those treatments successful once you leave the office. Your nurse is the one who will remind you to take the birth control pill with food so you don't throw up. She will offer sincere sympathy when your pregnancy test comes back negative again. The details and nuances that encompass a nurse's job are often overlooked and undervalued, but the benefit of a connection with the nurses at your doctor's office is tremendous.

To make the most of your connection with nurses, you should:

Be patient—It's not her fault if the doctor is slow getting into the room or the lab results took an extra day to arrive.

Be polite—Nurses understand that when you are hurting emotionally and physically you might not be at your best. However, being as polite as you can helps your time spent with them to be more comfortable.

Say thank you—A little gratitude goes a long way.

MENTAL-HEALTH PROFESSIONALS

Because body and mind are so connected, the goal of total wellness is to have balance and health in both. A psychologist or counselor can assist you in working through emotional struggles related to PCOS.

Going back to the CEO analogy, working with a therapist is like having a conflict-resolution team and knowledge manager in one. Resistance to change is often an internal conflict resulting from fear. A therapist can help you explore that fear and make sense of multiple sources of information to reduce fear and gain insight. Less resistance means that you can clear the way for motivation in order to make real progress. Resentment grows from unmet expectations. Once you work through these issues and achieve insight, your therapist will help you explore ways to apply this knowledge where it is needed most.

If you suffer from depression or anxiety to the point that your daily activities are affected, then a therapist is a must-have on your dream team. Because PCOS is a lifelong syndrome, new challenges may come up as you age. It's perfectly fine to have a therapist you can call on when things are tough. Sometimes all you need is a session or two to get back on track. Sometimes you need more time, which is perfectly fine. There is no need to suffer. Emotional health still takes work, but if it is a challenge, a therapist can ensure that your efforts are streamlined.

To get the best results from therapy, you should:

Say so if you don't like your therapist—It's okay. We don't take it personally. Healing is hinged on having a connection with your therapist, so if you don't like her, then find someone you do like to get the best outcome. That's not to say that your therapist won't make you mad or challenge you to grow, but there must be a rapport there to get the best from those challenging moments.

Be on time—Your therapist is dedicating an hour to work with you one-on-one. Being late is hurting your progress because it's hard to get through the therapeutic process in a shorter amount of time.

Reconsider canceling your appointment—Your desire to cancel may just be resistance. Are you sure you're too busy? Or perhaps you didn't like the way you felt in the last session.

Understand that you might feel worse before you get better—Sometimes therapy involves a lot of "unpacking" of beliefs and behaviors. The relief of insight might come later, but it will happen.

Do your homework—Those activities that your therapist gives you are not fluff. The goal of homework in therapy is to bridge the gap between the therapy session and real life. It is also meant to expand and reinforce what you're working on in sessions, without the time limitation.

Understand that therapists don't give advice—Should you leave your job? Divorce your spouse? Your therapist won't tell you, but she can help you explore the question from all the angles so you can make the most informed decision.

Understand that that issue you definitely don't want to talk about is probably the one you should bring up—Don't hold back. Therapists have heard everything.

Understand that your therapist takes privacy very seriously—She likely won't acknowledge you if you see her in town. She's not talking about you with her friends.

Understand that therapists don't prescribe medication—Medication is not a substitute for doing the work, but if your issue is more severe or is not responding well to therapy, you and your therapist can talk about connecting with your doctor or a psychiatrist. Sometimes medication can help you get to a point where therapy can start to work, and then you can consider coming off a medication. But do so only under a psychiatrist's care.

PHYSICAL THERAPISTS

If you have chronic pain, then a physical therapist is your secret weapon. Physical therapists are trained to reduce pain and restore mobility. Depending on what state you live in, you may not even need a referral from your doctor; however, it is always helpful to ensure that all of your providers are aware of one another.

To get the best results from working with a physical therapist, you should:

Be on time—This is a given when you're in any professional situation, but it's even more so for physical therapists. Each physical-therapy session is structured and planned out. If you're late, you run the risk of cutting into that plan, which only hurts your progress in the long run.

Avoid distractions—Turn off your cell phone, and, if possible, find alternative care for your children (if you have any).

Keep in mind that getting physical therapy is an active process—It isn't passive like getting a massage. You are very often an active participant in the process.

Share your medical history with your physical therapist—The physical pain you are in might be caused by an issue somewhere else in your body. To get the most efficient care, be sure to give your physical therapist a full history of your injury or condition. If it is difficult to talk about (for example, a postop or traumatic injury), then consider writing it down. This helps your physical therapist provide targeted care.

Do your homework—Your physical therapist will give you exercises to do at home. Often, the physical-therapy sessions are more to diagnose, evaluate, and introduce treatments. The responsibility for long-term change falls on what you do *outside* of the office. Doing the prescribed exercises consistently will shorten treatment time and improve the outcome.

Be willing to work through the pain—Keep in mind that while the goal is less pain, sometimes there is more discomfort in the treatments. If this happens, be sure to tell your physical therapist, but understand that it is often pain with a purpose. Taking your pain medication as prescribed can help you manage the discomfort that might come up as a result of the therapy.

Understand that progress may not be straightforward—Sometimes it is a case of two steps forward, one step back. If you have concerns about your progress, be sure to ask.

SIGNIFICANT OTHERS

If you are married, then you have a wonderful support system built right in! The trick is to express your needs in a way that is effective and brings you closer together as a couple. Generally, when communicating with your spouse, it's better to not begin statements with pronouncements about what they should do or what you think they do—what we call *you-statements*. The problem with you-statements is that the person on the receiving end of a you-statement can wind up feeling defensive ("Why do *you* always . . ." "*You*'re so . . .") long before they've even been told what exactly you're feeling and why you're feeling it. At best, you-statements tend to leave couples revisiting the same argument over and over. On the other hand, I-statements provide a lot of information ("When this happens, *I* feel . . ." "*I* prefer when . . .") before bringing the other person's responsibility into it. Ideally, your I-statement also offers a solution that leaves the matter open for either agreement or more discussion.

Consider the following examples of some potentially tricky interactions and how you can avoid destructive accusations by using I-statements, which promote healthy, productive interaction:

Accusation—"You always bring home junk food!"
I-statement—"I'm trying really hard to stay away from sugar, and it would help me manage cravings better if it weren't in the house. Can you enjoy junk food outside of the house?"

Accusation—"You never listen to me when I try to talk about my PCOS."
I-statement—"It would help me feel less anxious if I could talk about my doctor's appointment with you."

How much information does your partner need? At first, they need just enough to know that your symptoms are real. When you start talking about having kids, then it's a team effort, from the doctor's visits to being a shoulder to cry on if you need it.

When it comes to infertility, the two of you are in this together. I strongly recommend that your partner accompany you to doctors' visits as often as possible. Not only does it provide you with support during stressful times, but it also gives your partner a clearly defined role as your support system. Give your partner a job during appointments—like taking notes on the doctor's recommendations. Doing so will help your partner feel useful and encourage attentive participation.

It is very possible for the PCOS to bring you and your partner closer together. When any couple faces a challenge, they have two options: to move toward one another or to insulate themselves and move away from one another. A lot of factors come into play here: personality type, conflict style, and willingness to invest in the relationship. There are some people who hit PCOS as the first bump in the relationship road, and it's the beginning of the end. Then there are other people who take a very real relationship challenge and get closer.

One of the best ways to boost your relationship is to be intentional in the way you communicate with your partner. There are communication patterns that can make or break your relationship. Coping with a chronic syndrome like PCOS will bring out less-than-stellar communication patterns in a hurry. Whenever you communicate with your partner, it's important to evaluate it by asking yourself, *Did that exchange bring me closer to my partner or put distance between us?*

According to renowned psychiatrist and psychotherapist William Glasser, these seven communication patterns are poison to any relationship:

1. *Nagging*—This unfortunate style can manifest in either partner. Perhaps your partner is constantly reminding you to exercise more. Or you may find yourself pushing your partner to attend all of your doctor's appointments.
2. *Blaming*—This is heartbreaking when it comes to infertility. Very often women blame themselves enough without the additional blame. If your partner is blaming you for your infertility, acne, or any other PCOS-related symptom, stop what you're doing and make an appointment with a qualified therapist.
3. *Criticizing*—Finding fault in anything and everything is counterproductive. These kinds of critiques are not shared in a way that is beneficial to the final outcome.
4. *Complaining*—This is a very common communication pattern. Many people have no idea of the impact their complaining has on loved ones. When it comes to PCOS, there is plenty to complain about; however, continually complaining to your spouse can be exhausting and leave them feeling powerless. Instead, communicate what you *need*, and move forward.
5. *Threatening*—Threatening to leave, to withhold affection, or even to choose to remain childless (with the intent of hurting the other person) is toxic to a relationship.
6. *Bribing or rewarding to control*—This approach ensures that you will keep problem interactions on repeat. Nothing gets solved with this approach. You can be guaranteed that whatever problem you're attempting to control with bribing or rewarding will show up again.
7. *Punishing*—Physical fights are never okay. Name calling and other verbal attacks are not helpful.

Conversely, Glasser outlines seven relationship-building communication patterns:

1. *Supporting*—Your spouse can support your efforts to eat healthily and exercise. They can also support you in doctor visits, reminding you to take your medication, and so forth.

2. *Encouraging*—This is a tricky one. It should actually be used more sparingly than you might think. Your spouse can encourage you to keep going if you express that your motivation is falling apart. The difficulty is that occasionally it turns an ugly corner and begins to feel like nagging. And sometimes it's time to discuss taking a break from interventions or to try something different.

3. *Listening*—This is an incredibly helpful communication pattern. Active listening includes listening while making eye contact (no cell phones allowed!). The secret to active listening is reflecting. Your listener should hear what you have to say and then accurately rephrase it. There is nothing that makes you feel more understood or validated than having your ideas reflected back. Sometimes a person will make an effort to reflect and get it totally wrong. It's okay to gently correct their attempt and explain again.

4. *Accepting*—This one is important for those of us with PCOS. In fact, it is the one thing we struggle with and the one thing we want most in the world from our significant others. To have someone hear you, understand, and accept is a blessing and relief.

5. *Trusting*—We have to be able to trust our spouses to keep our medical challenges quiet. This is a nonnegotiable. Nothing should be shared with anyone without your consent. Not with your parents, not with his parents, and certainly not on social media.

6. *Respecting*—This is where good communication at the outset can be helpful. While PCOS has physical manifestations, it is largely an unseen challenge. If your spouse understands your challenge, respect becomes much easier.

7. *Negotiating differences*—There are many different ways to manage PCOS, so this is essential. You may prefer more natural solutions, whereas your partner might be more comfortable with medical interventions. You may deeply ache to have your own children while your spouse is comfortable with adoption. Talk about these differences; bring them out into the open.[2]

If you are having trouble with your communication patterns, it's not a deal-breaker or a lost cause. We often bring to our relationships the patterns we learned growing up. It's neither a failure nor an attack on your parents. We are all doing the best we know how in any situation. If you're struggling, it may be a sign that more support is needed. I strongly recommend that you ask for help before the unwanted communication patterns become a well-established habit. The right therapist can help you gain insight into your communication style and develop a style that brings you and your spouse closer.

JOURNAL QUESTIONS

1. What do you need from your doctor?
2. Who are the people on your wellness dream team?
3. What do you need from your significant other when it comes to your health and well-being? Is that something they can do?
4. What's one communication pattern you want to change? How will you do it?

12

Going Forward

Having a chronic condition like PCOS can seem overwhelming. There is an initial learning curve following diagnosis, but over time you become the expert in being the healthiest version of yourself.

PCOS is not a disability; it is simply a condition that may make you have to take a different approach to your overall health. There's clarity and ease in knowing what works for your body and what doesn't. We know that the common diet and exercise recommendations aren't always a good fit for us. The beautiful thing is that this gives you the opportunity to design an approach to wellness that is both unique and authentic.

Suffering doesn't come from the diagnosis; it comes from how we respond to the diagnosis. From this moment forward you have a choice about how you want to thrive with PCOS. By embracing PCOS, you have the leverage to change the outcome of your long-term health.

Here, at the end of the book, I'm issuing you a challenge. One of the most common ways to self-sabotage is to keep searching for a solution, but the bottom line is that *you* are the solution. It's time to stop searching and start doing. You know what you need to do. Trust yourself to make it happen.

IMPLEMENTING YOUR LIFESTYLE STRATEGY

Start with small, simple goals. Motivation and willpower are only as strong as your hardest day, so be sure to use that as your starting point. If it feels good to do more, then that's okay. What cardio exercise will you do for at least ten minutes every day? Evaluate your plan every month—or more if you are feeling bored or like you've hit a plateau.

Decide how you're going to change your diet. What times of day are easier for you and harder to stay on plan? Figure out how to make changes during those times that diet is a challenge. Remember to stay hydrated.

How will you manage stress? Mindfulness meditation isn't nearly as far off as it sounds, although taking a walk outside or even simply breathing deeply are often helpful.

What medical interventions do you need? Make an appointment with your doctor if you have questions or if it's been a while since you have seen her.

If you're not sleeping well, what will you change to ensure that you get seven to eight hours every night? Nothing is more important than your health. Focus on making the hour before bedtime a nonnegotiable screen-free time to settle down and transition to sleep time.

When you're deciding what to implement first, it's helpful to use the 80/20 rule. What is the strategy that you can implement first that will give you the most progress, the most satisfaction, or the most healing for your effort? Once you've mastered the change that brings the most benefit, you can add to it with smaller strategies.

Implement. Evaluate. Adjust if necessary. Repeat.

This is the strategy for life. You will develop a familiarity with lifestyle strategies that you have never felt before. Over time, this ability will expand to all parts of your life. You are at the beginning of your defining moment. How you choose to manage your PCOS will affect every aspect of your life. It may seem like a challenge that is insurmountable, but, I assure you, the success is found in the decisions you make from one moment to the next.

Understand that balance is a verb. It's not a destination. It's an ongoing mind-set to maintain awareness of the internal accounting of energy being given and energy coming in. Throughout your day, your life, holidays, and life changes, your health is first.

Review your wins. Progress isn't always on the scale. Sometimes a win is realizing that you feel more confident in social situations. Or perhaps you realize you've forgotten about your anxiety for a few days. Any time you choose to treat yourself well, any time you eat healthily, whenever you remember to manage your stress . . . all of those count as wins, and it's important to acknowledge those wins on a daily basis.

Life is your canvas. You have an infinite number of colors to choose from as you create your masterpiece. Sometimes there are elements on the canvas you didn't put there, but they're beautiful all the same. You may not realize this, but having PCOS can be a remarkable part of the picture you are creating right now, even if you're struggling at the moment. Your success story is in the making. Release any doubt that you can make healthy changes.

This is a call to heal not only your body but also your mind. Healing from PCOS is not a quick fix. It is a lifelong process of gently and accurately nurturing your body. By adding the missing piece of mind-set, you are well on your way to transforming motivation into lasting results. Not every day will be perfect. Not every choice will be ideal. However, by gently maintaining your focus on your health, you'll learn as you go, your overall health will improve, and you will thrive as a woman with PCOS.

Notes

CHAPTER 1

1. Jacqueline Boyle and Helena J. Teede, "Polycystic Ovary Syndrome: An Update," *Australian Family Physician* 41, no. 10 (2012): 752–56, http://www.racgp .org.au/afp/2012/october/polycystic-ovary-syndrome/.

2. Ibid.

3. Michael L. Traub, "Assessing and Treating Insulin Resistance in Women with Polycystic Ovarian Syndrome," *World Journal of Diabetes* 2, no. 3 (2011): 33–40, https://www.wjgnet.com/1948-9358/full/v2/i3/33.htm.

4. Susan Sam, "Obesity and Polycystic Ovary Syndrome," *Obesity Management* 3, no. 2 (2007): 69–73, https://www.ncbi.nlm.nih.gov/pmc/articles/ PMC2861983/.

5. Andrea Dunaif, "Insulin Resistance and the Polycystic Ovary Syndrome: Mechanism and Implications for Pathogenesis," *Endocrine Reviews* 18, no. 6 (1997): 774–800, https://academic.oup.com/edrv/article-lookup/doi/10.1210/ edrv.18.6.0318.

6. Fiona McCulloch, "Does PCOS Make Your Brain More Hungry?" White Lotus Naturopathic Clinic and Integrated Health (website), July 22, 2014, http:// www.whitelotusclinic.ca/blog/dr-fiona-nd/hunger-pcos-brain-insulin/.

7. Samantha K. Hutchison, Nigel K. Stepto, Cheryce L. Harrison, Lisa J. Moran, Boyd J. Strauss, and Helena J. Teede, "Effects of Exercise on Insulin Resistance and Body Composition in Overweight and Obese Women with and without Polycystic Ovary Syndrome," *Journal of Clinical Endocrinology and Metabolism* 96, no. 1 (2011): E48–56, https://academic.oup.com/jcem/article-lookup/ doi/10.1210/jc.2010-0828.

8. Olga T. Hardy, Michael P. Czech, and Silvia Corvera, "What Causes the Insulin Resistance Underlying Obesity?" *Current Opinion in Endocrinology, Diabetes, and Obesity* 19, no. 2 (2012): 81–87, https://www.ncbi.nlm.nih.gov/pmc/articles/PMC4038351/.

9. Angela, "What Happens to Women with PCOS as They Age?" PCOS Nutrition Center, January 23, 2016, http://www.pcosnutrition.com/aging/.

CHAPTER 2

1. Siobhan E. McCluskey, J. Hubert Lacey, and J. M. Pearce, "Binge-Eating and Polycystic Ovaries," *The Lancet* 340, no. 8821 (1992): 723.

2. American Heart Association, "Saturated Fats," Healthy for Good (website), last updated March 24, 2017, https://healthyforgood.heart.org/Eat-smart/Articles/Saturated-Fats.

3. Visit http://allrecipes.com.

4. Rebecca L. Thomson, Simon Spedding, and Jonathan D. Buckley, "Vitamin D in the Aetiology and Management of Polycystic Ovary Syndrome," *Clinical Endocrinology* 77, no. 3 (2012): 343–50.

5. John C. Mavropoulos, William S. Yancy, Juanita Hepburn, and Eric C. Westman, "The Effects of a Low-Carbohydrate, Ketogenic Diet on the Polycystic Ovary Syndrome: A Pilot Study," *Nutrition and Metabolism* 2 (2005): 35, https://www.ncbi.nlm.nih.gov/pmc/articles/PMC1334192/.

6. For more information on consuming a Paleo diet if you have a PCOS diagnosis, see Stephani Ruper, "Paleo and PCOS," *Paleo for Women* (blog), May 5, 2012, http://paleoforwomen.com/paleo-and-pcos/.

CHAPTER 4

1. Christina Boufis, "How Your Sleep Affects Your Heart," WebMD (website), 2011, accessed April 4, 2017, http://www.webmd.com/sleep-disorders/features/how-sleep-affects-your-heart#1.

2. Ananya Mandal, "What Is Ghrelin?" News Medical (website), last updated, September 17, 2014, http://www.news-medical.net/health/What-is-Ghrelin.aspx.

3. Pai C. Kao, Shu-Chu Shiesh, and Ta-Jen Wu, "Serum C-Reactive Protein as a Marker for Wellness Assessment," *Annals of Clinical and Laboratory Science* 36, no. 2 (Spring 2006): 163–69, http://www.annclinlabsci.org/content/36/2/163.full.

4. Larry Rosen, "Relax, Turn Off Your Phone, and Go to Sleep," *Harvard Business Review*, August 31, 2015, https://hbr.org/2015/08/research-shows-how-anxiety-and-technology-are-affecting-our-sleep.

5. Harris R. Lieberman, William J. Tharion, Barbara Shukitt-Hale, Karen L. Speckman, and Richard Tulley, "Effects of Caffeine, Sleep Loss, and Stress on Cognitive Performance and Mood during U.S. Navy SEAL Training," *Psychopharmacology* 164, no. 3 (2002): 250–61.

CHAPTER 5

1. National Institute of Mental Health, "Any Anxiety Disorder among Adults," National Institutes of Health, accessed April 19, 2017, https://www.nimh.nih.gov/health/statistics/prevalence/any-anxiety-disorder-among-adults.shtml.

2. American Psychological Association, "Anxiety," accessed April 7, 2017, http://www.apa.org/topics/anxiety/.

3. Judy G. McCook, Beth A. Bailey, Stacey L. Williams, Sheeba Anand, and Nancy E. Reame, "Differential Contributions of Polycystic Ovary Syndrome (PCOS) Manifestations to Psychological Symptoms," *Journal of Behavioral Health Services and Research* 42, no. 3 (2015): 383–94.

4. A. Rocco, P. Falaschi, G. Perrone, P. Pancheri, M. Rosa, and L. Zichella, "Psychoneuroendocrine Aspects of Polycystic Ovary Syndrome," *Journal of Psychosomatic Obstetrics and Gynecology* 12, no. 2 (1991): 169–79.

5. Beck Institute for Cognitive Behavior, "What Is Cognitive Behavior Therapy (CBT)?" BeckInstitute.org, accessed April 18, 2017, https://www.beckinstitute.org/get-informed/what-is-cognitive-therapy/.

6. National Institute of Mental Health, "Any Anxiety Disorder."

7. Charles S. Lieber, "Alcohol: Its Metabolism and Interaction with Nutrients," *Annual Review of Nutrition* 20 (2000): 395–430.

8. Faranak Sharifi, Sahar Mazloomi, Reza Hajihosseini, and Saideh Mazloomzadeh, "Serum Magnesium Concentrations in Polycystic Ovary Syndrome and Its Association with Insulin Resistance," *Gynecological Endocrinology* 28, no. 1 (2012): 7–11.

9. Dr. Axe [Josh Axe], "Top 10 Magnesium Rich Foods Plus Proven Benefits," accessed April 23, 2017, https://draxe.com/magnesium-deficient-top-10-magnesium-rich-foods-must-eating/.

10. Michael Otto and Jasper A. J. Smits, *Exercise for Mood and Anxiety: Proven Strategies for Overcoming Depression and Enhancing Well-Being* (New York: Oxford University Press, 2011).

11. Jon Vøllestad, Børge Sivertsen, and Geir Høstmark Nielsen, "Mindfulness-Based Stress Reduction for Patients with Anxiety Disorders: Evaluation in a Randomized Controlled Trial," *Behavior Research and Therapy* 49, no. 4 (2011): 281–88, http://www.sciencedirect.com/science/article/pii/S0005796711000246.

12. John R. Hughes, "Psychological Effects of Habitual Aerobic Exercise: A Critical Review," *Preventive Medicine* 13, no. 1 (1986): 66–78.

13. Shelley Taylor, "Coping Strategies," in collaboration with the Psychosocial Working Group, MacArthur Research Network on Socioeconomic Status and Health (website), last revised July 1998, http://www.macses.ucsf.edu/research/psychosocial/coping.php.

CHAPTER 6

1. Deborah S. Hasin, Renee D. Goodwin, Frederick S. Stinson, and Bridget F. Grant, "Epidemiology of Major Depressive Disorder: Results from the National Epidemiologic Survey on Alcoholism and Related Conditions," *Archives of General Psychiatry* 62, no. 10 (2005): 1097–1106, http://jamanetwork.com/journals/jamapsychiatry/fullarticle/208965.

2. National Institute of Health, "Dysthymic Disorder among Adults," accessed May 12, 2017, https://www.nimh.nih.gov/health/statistics/prevalence/dysthymic-disorder-among-adults.shtml.

3. Anxiety and Depression Association of America, "Depression: Understand the Facts," accessed May 12, 2017, https://www.adaa.org/understanding-anxiety/depression.

4. You can get help from the Suicide Prevention Lifeline at its website, https://suicidepreventionlifeline.org, or by calling 1-800-723-8255.

5. National Institute of Child Health and Human Development, "Are There Disorders or Conditions Associated with PCOS?" accessed May 11, 2017, https://www.nichd.nih.gov/health/topics/PCOS/conditioninfo/Pages/conditions-associated.aspx.

6. For example, Sue Pearson, Mike Schmidt, George Patton, Terry Dwyer, Leigh Blizzard, Petr Otahal, and Alison Venn, "Depression and Insulin Resistance: Cross-Sectional Associations in Young Adults," *Diabetes Care* 33, no. 5 (2010): 1128–33, https://doi.org/10.2337/dc09-1940.

7. Ibid.

8. Natalie Rasgon and Shana Elman, "When Not to Treat Depression in PCOS with Antidepressants," *Current Psychiatry* 4, no. 2 (February 2005): 47–60, http://www.mdedge.com/currentpsychiatry/article/66214/depression/when-not-treat-depression-pcos-antidepressants.

9. Margarita Tartakovsky, "Top Relapse Triggers for Depression and How to Prevent Them," Psych Central (website), last reviewed July 17, 2016, https://psychcentral.com/lib/top-relapse-triggers-for-depression-how-to-prevent-them/.

CHAPTER 7

1. Guy Winch, "Why We All Need to Practice Emotional First Aid," filmed November 7, 2014, TEDxLinnaeusUniversity video, 17:24, https://www.ted.com/talks/guy_winch_the_case_for_emotional_hygiene.

2. John M. Grohol, "15 Common Cognitive Distortions," *Psych Central* (website), 2016, accessed April 20, 2017, https://psychcentral.com/lib/15-common -cognitive-distortions/.

3. Winch, "Why We All Need to Practice Emotional First Aid."

CHAPTER 8

1. Eric J. Nestler, Steven E. Hyman, David A. Holtzman, and Robert C. Malenka, eds., "Neural and Neuroendocrine Control of the Internal Milieu," in *Molecular Neuropharmacology: A Foundation for Clinical Neuroscience*, 248–59 (New York: McGraw-Hill Medical, 2009).

2. D. K. Virsaladze, K. Natmeladze, I. Topuria, A. Natmeladze, and N. Paichadze, "The Effect of Dopamine on Neuroendocrine Disorders in Women with PCOS under Chronic Stress Conditions," *Endocrine Abstracts* 11 (2006): P597.

3. American Institute of Stress, "The Holmes-Rahe Stress Inventory," accessed April 23, 2017, https://www.stress.org/holmes-rahe-stress-inventory/.

4. Originally published as Neil B. Kavey, "Stress and Insomnia," *sleepmatters* (Spring 2001), available online at https://sleepfoundation.org/ask-the-expert/ stress-and-insomnia/.

5. Ljudmila Stojanovich and Dragomir Marisavljevich, "Stress as a Trigger of Autoimmune Disease," *Autoimmunity Reviews* 7, no. 3 (2008): 209–13.

6. Madhav Goyal, Sonal Singh, Erica M. S. Sibinga, Neda F. Gould, Anastasia Rowland-Seymour, Ritu Sharma, Zackary Berger, Dana Sleicher, David D. Maron, Hasan M. Shihab, Padmini D. Ranasinghe, Shauna Linn, Shonali Saha, Eric B. Bass, and Jennifer A. Haythornthwaite, "Meditation Programs for Psychological Stress and Well-Being: A Systematic Review and Meta-analysis," *JAMA Internal Medicine* 174, no. 3 (2014): 357–68.

7. Antoni J. Duleba and Anuja Dokras, "Is PCOS an Inflammatory Process?" *Fertility and Sterility* 97, no 1 (2012): 7–12, http://www.fertstert.org/article/ S0015-0282(11)02799-3/fulltext.

CHAPTER 9

1. Nazia Raja-Khan, Katrina Agito, Julie Shah, Christy M. Stetter, Theresa S. Gustafson, Holly Socolow, Allen R. Kunselman, Diane K. Reibel, and Richard S. Legro, "Mindfulness-Based Stress Reduction for Overweight/Obese Women with and without Polycystic Ovary Syndrome: Design and Methods of a Pilot Randomized Controlled Trial," *Contemporary Clinical Trials* 41 (2015): 287–97.

2. Thich Nhat Hanh, "Five Steps to Mindfulness," Mindful (website), August 23, 2010, https://www.mindful.org/five-steps-to-mindfulness/.

3. Robert A. Emmons and Michael E. McCullough, "Counting Blessings versus Burdens: An Experimental Investigation of Gratitude and Subjective Well-Being in Daily Life," *Journal of Personality and Social Psychology* 84, no. 2 (2003): 377–89.

4. Madhav Goyal, Sonal Singh, Erica M. S. Sibinga, Neda F. Gould, Anastasia Rowland-Seymour, Ritu Sharma, Zackary Berger, Dana Sleicher, David D. Maron, Hasan M. Shihab, Padmini D. Ranasinghe, Shauna Linn, Shonali Saha, Eric B. Bass, and Jennifer A. Haythornthwaite, "Meditation Programs for Psychological Stress and Well-Being: A Systematic Review and Meta-analysis," *JAMA Internal Medicine* 174, no. 3 (2014): 357–68.

5. F. Zeidan, J. A. Grant, C. A. Brown, J. G. McHaffie, and R. C. Coghill, "Mindfulness Meditation–Related Pain Relief: Evidence for Unique Brain Mechanisms in the Regulation of Pain," *Neuroscience Letters* 520, no. 2 (2012): 165–73.

6. Jon Kabat-Zinn, *Wherever You Go, There You Are: Mindfulness Meditation for Everyday Life* (New York: Hyperion, 1994).

CHAPTER 10

1. Gavneet K. Pruthi and Nandita Babu, "Physical and Psychosocial Impact of Acne in Adult Females," *Indian Journal of Dermatology* 57, no. 1 (2012): 26–29, http://www.e-ijd.org/article.asp?issn=0019-5154;year=2012;volume=57;issue=1; spage=26;epage=29;aulast=Pruthi. And see Cornelia Kean, "New Survey Highlights Emotional Toll of Adult Acne," *The Dermatologist* 16, no. 8 (2008), http://www.the-dermatologist.com/article/9048.

2. Deepani Rathnayake and Rodney Sinclair, "Innovative Use of Spironolactone as an Antiandrogen in the Treatment of Female Pattern Hair Loss," *Dermatologic Clinics* 28, no. 3 (2010): 611–18.

3. Tobechi L. Ebede, Emily L. Arch, and Diane Berson. "Hormonal Treatment of Acne in Women," *Journal of Clinical and Aesthetic Dermatology* 2, no. 12 (2009): 16–22, https://www.ncbi.nlm.nih.gov/pmc/articles/PMC2923944/.

4. Daisy Kopera, Elisabeth Wehr, and Barbara Obermayer-Pietsch, "Endocrinology of Hirsutism," *International Journal of Trichology* 2, no. 1 (2010): 30–35, http://www.ijtrichology.com/article.asp?issn=0974-7753;year=2010;volume=2;is sue=1;spage=30;epage=35;aulast=Kopera.

5. Molly Quinn, Kanade Shinkai, Lauri Pasch, Lili Kuzmich, Marcelle Cedars, and Heather Huddleston, "Prevalence of Androgenic Alopecia in Patients with Polycystic Ovary Syndrome and Characterization of Associated Clinical and Biochemical Features," *Fertility and Sterility* 101, no. 4 (2014): 1129–34, http://www.fertstert.org/article/S0015-0282(14)00033-8/fulltext.

6. Advanced Fertility Center of Chicago, "Ovulation Problems and Infertility: Treatment of Ovulation Problems with Clomid and Other Fertility Drugs," accessed April 3, 2017, http://www.advancedfertility.com/inducovu.htm.

7. *Drugs.com*, "Gonadotropins," last updated June 6, 2017, accessed May 15, 2017, https://www.drugs.com/drug-class/gonadotropins.html.

8. Society for Endocrinology, "Luteinising Hormone," *You and Your Hormones* (website), last updated January 7, 2015, http://www.yourhormones.info/hormones/luteinising_hormone.aspx.

9. Maria Masters, "12 Facts You Should Know about Ovarian Cysts," *Health.com*, 2015, Accessed May 15, 2017. http://www.health.com/health/gallery/0,,20955242,00.html/view-all.

10. Aria Pearson, "Youthful Infertility Balanced by Late-Blooming Ovaries," *New Scientist*, February 25, 2009, https://www.newscientist.com/article/mg20126973-700-youthful-infertility-balanced-by-late-blooming-ovaries/.

CHAPTER 11

1. Carol Peckham, "Medscape Physician Compensation Report 2016," Medscape (website), April 1, 2016, http://www.medscape.com/features/slideshow/compensation/2016/public/overview.

2. William Glasser Institute–US, "Choice Theory," WGlasser.com, accessed April 2, 2017, http://www.wglasser.com/the-glasser-approach/choice-theory.

Glossary

anxiety A mental-health issue characterized by worry or fear to the point that it disrupts daily life.

binge eating Consuming a large amount of food in a short amount of time, typically as a coping strategy. Can reach severity to be considered an eating disorder.

body mass index (BMI) A way of estimating body fat based on height and weight. Not accurate, but often used because of its convenience.

cortisol Has many functions in the body: allows for higher blood sugar, which can lead to insulin resistance and inflammation—especially significant for women with PCOS. Commonly known as the *stress hormone.*

C-reactive protein (CRP) A chemical produced by the liver that increases with disease or inflammation in the body.

depression Depending on the cause, an emotional issue or brain disorder resulting in a consistently depressed mood or loss of interest in activities. Can severely impact daily life.

diuretic Any substance or medication promoting water loss and increased urine production.

electrolysis A method of hair removal where a tiny probe is inserted into the hair follicle and either chemicals or heat are used to stop future growth. Time consuming because only one hair at a time can be treated; however, it is permanent.

emotional hygiene Being aware of our psychological wellness and mindfully addressing it with short habits built into the daily routine.

equifinality The principle that within any framework there can be many ways to reach the same result.

estrogen A hormone in the body produced by the ovaries and body fat. Controls the menstrual cycle and promotes health in many areas of the body, including the heart, bones, and brain.

follicle A small gland or sac. Hair comes out of a hair follicle. The ovaries have follicles that are fluid-filled sacs that hold an egg. The egg is released from the follicle when it is mature; however, in women with PCOS, the eggs might not reach maturity to be released, due to hormonal imbalances.

glycemic index (GI) A ranking of carbohydrates from 0 to 100 according to how much they spike blood sugar after eating.

hypothalamic-pituitary-adrenal axis (HPA axis) A system in the body that controls reactions to stress as well as immunity, digestion, and mood.

insulin resistance A condition where the body's cells don't respond to insulin's attempt to get sugar into the cells. This leads to higher levels of sugar (glucose) in the blood stream.

macronutrients (macros) The nutrients that the body needs in large amounts. Generally broken down into fat, protein, and carbohydrates.

major depressive disorder (MDD) Characterized by low mood or lack of enjoyment in normal activities for at least two weeks. Also known as *clinical depression.*

mindfulness-based cognitive therapy (MBCT) A blend of mindfulness practices, meditation, and cognitive therapy. Designed to help people who have chronic bouts of depression.

mindfulness-based stress reduction (MBSR) A program that helps people manage pain and stress by focusing on the present moment.

persistent depressive disorder (PDD) Characterized by low mood and other symptoms of depression lasting for over two years. Also known as *dysthymia.*

polycystic ovary syndrome (PCOS) A collection of symptoms caused by the way a woman's body responds to androgens and insulin. Typical symptoms include no ovulation or infrequent ovulation, elevated testosterone levels that can result in hirsutism, and/or male-pattern hair loss, and acne, along with multiple cysts on the ovaries.

progesterone A hormone produced in the ovaries that has many functions, including maintaining pregnancy and libido. Also plays a part in maintaining monthly menstrual cycles.

rumination From a psychological perspective, the process of repetitively going over a problem or worry without coming to a conclusion of some sort. Can lead to anxiety and depression.

serotonin A chemical made in the body that is responsible for stabilizing mood. A neurotransmitter derived from tryptophan. Also known as the *happiness hormone.*

testosterone Commonly known as a male hormone or androgen, it is a naturally occurring hormone in women as well. Testosterone is made by the ovaries and adrenal glands. Testosterone levels are often elevated in women with PCOS.

tryptophan An amino acid supplied by eating foods such as turkey, eggs, cheese, and nuts.

Bibliography

Advanced Fertility Center of Chicago. "Ovulation Problems and Infertility: Treatment of Ovulation Problems with Clomid and Other Fertility Drugs." Accessed April 3, 2017. http://www.advancedfertility.com/inducovu.htm.

American Heart Association. "Saturated Fats." Healthy for Good (website). Last updated March 24, 2017. https://healthyforgood.heart.org/Eat-smart/Articles/Saturated-Fats.

American Institute of Stress. "The Holmes-Rahe Stress Inventory." Accessed April 23, 2017. https://www.stress.org/holmes-rahe-stress-inventory/.

American Psychological Association. "Anxiety." Accessed April 7, 2017. http://www.apa.org/topics/anxiety/.

Angela. "What Happens to Women with PCOS as They Age?" PCOS Nutrition Center. January 23, 2016. http://www.pcosnutrition.com/aging/.

Anxiety and Depression Association of America. Depression: Understand the Facts." Accessed May 12, 2017. https://www.adaa.org/understanding-anxiety/depression.

Azziz, Ricardo. "Diagnosis of Polycystic Ovarian Syndrome: The Rotterdam Criteria Are Premature." *Journal of Clinical Endocrinology and Metabolism* 91, no. 3 (2006): 781–85. https://academic.oup.com/jcem/article-lookup/doi/10.1210/jc.2005-2153.

Barnard L., D. Ferriday, N. Guenther, B. Strauss, A. H. Balen, and L. Dye. "Quality of Life and Psychological Well Being in Polycystic Ovary Syndrome." *Human Reproduction* 22, no. 8 (2007): 2279–86. https://academic.oup.com/humrep/article-lookup/doi/10.1093/humrep/dem108.

Barr, Suezanne, Sue Reeves, Kay Sharp, and Yvonne M. Jeanes. "An Isocaloric Low Glycemic Index Diet Improves Insulin Sensitivity in Women with Polycystic Ovary Syndrome." *Journal of the Academy of Nutrition and Dietetics* 113, no. 11 (2013): 1523–31.

Beck Institute for Cognitive Behavior. "What Is Cognitive Behavior Therapy (CBT)?" BeckInstitute.org. Accessed April 18, 2017. https://www.beckinstitute.org/get-informed/what-is-cognitive-therapy/.

Boufis, Christina. "How Your Sleep Affects Your Heart." WebMD (website). 2011. Accessed April 4, 2017. http://www.webmd.com/sleep-disorders/features/how-sleep-affects-your-heart#1.

Boyle, Jacqueline, and Helena J. Teede. "Polycystic Ovary Syndrome: An Update." *Australian Family Physician* 41, no. 10 (2012): 752–56. http://www.racgp.org.au/afp/2012/october/polycystic-ovary-syndrome/.

Caffeine Informer (website). "Caffeine Metabolism." Last modified August 28, 2016. https://www.caffeineinformer.com/caffeine-metabolism.

Costantino, D., G. Minozzi, F. Minozzi, and C. Guaraldi. "Metabolic and Hormonal Effects of Myo-inositol in Women with Polycystic Ovary Syndrome: A Double-Blind Trial." *European Review for Medical and Pharmacological Sciences* 13, no. 2 (2009): 105–10. http://www.europeanreview.org/wp/wp-content/uploads/604.pdf.

Dr. Axe [Josh Axe]. "Top 10 Magnesium Rich Foods Plus Proven Benefits." Accessed April 23, 2017. https://draxe.com/magnesium-deficient-top-10-magnesium-rich-foods-must-eating/.

Drugs.com. "Gonadotropins." Last updated June 6, 2017. Accessed May 15, 2017. https://www.drugs.com/drug-class/gonadotropins.html.

Duleba, Antoni J., and Anuja Dokras. "Is PCOS an Inflammatory Process?" *Fertility and Sterility* 97, no. 1 (2012): 7–12. http://www.fertstert.org/article/S0015-0282(11)02799-3/fulltext.

Dunaif, Andrea. "Insulin Resistance and the Polycystic Ovary Syndrome: Mechanism and Implications for Pathogenesis." *Endocrine Reviews* 18, no. 6 (1997): 774–800. https://academic.oup.com/edrv/article-lookup/doi/10.1210/edrv.18.6.0318.

Ebede, Tobechi L., Emily L. Arch, and Diane Berson. "Hormonal Treatment of Acne in Women." *Journal of Clinical and Aesthetic Dermatology* 2, no. 12 (2009): 16–22. https://www.ncbi.nlm.nih.gov/pmc/articles/PMC2923944/.

Emmons, Robert A., and Michael E. McCullough. "Counting Blessings versus Burdens: An Experimental Investigation of Gratitude and Subjective Well-Being in Daily Life." *Journal of Personality and Social Psychology* 84, no. 2 (2003): 377–89.

Escobar-Morreale, H. F., E. Carmina, D. Dewailly, A. Gambineri, F. Kelestimur, P. Moghetti, M. Pugeat, J. Qiao, C. N. Wijeyaratne, S. F. Witchel, and R. J. Norman. "Epidemiology, Diagnosis and Management of Hirsutism: A Consensus Statement by the Androgen Excess and Polycystic Ovary Syndrome Society." *Human Reproduction Update* 19, no. 2 (2012): 146–70. https://academic.oup.com/humupd/article/19/2/207/583370/Epidemiology-diagnosis-and-management-of-hirsutism.

Goyal, Madhav, Sonal Singh, Erica M. S. Sibinga, Neda F. Gould, Anastasia Rowland-Seymour, Ritu Sharma, Zackary Berger, Dana Sleicher, David D. Maron, Hasan M. Shihab, Padmini D. Ranasinghe, Shauna Linn, Shonali Saha, Eric B. Bass, and Jennifer A. Haythornthwaite. "Meditation Programs for Psychological Stress and Well-Being: A Systematic Review and Meta-analysis." *JAMA Internal Medicine* 174, no. 3 (2014): 357–68.

Grohol, John M. "15 Common Cognitive Distortions." *Psych Central* (website). 2016. Accessed April 20, 2017. https://psychcentral.com/lib/15-common-cognitive-distortions/.

Hardy, Olga T., Michael P. Czech, and Silvia Corvera. "What Causes the Insulin Resistance Underlying Obesity?" *Current Opinion in Endocrinology, Diabetes, and Obesity* 19, no. 2 (2012): 81–87. https://www.ncbi.nlm.nih.gov/pmc/articles/PMC4038351/.

Hasin, Deborah S., Renee D. Goodwin, Frederick S. Stinson, and Bridget F. Grant. "Epidemiology of Major Depressive Disorder: Results from the National Epidemiologic Survey on Alcoholism and Related Conditions." *Archives of General Psychiatry* 62, no. 10 (2005): 1097–1106. http://jamanetwork.com/journals/jamapsychiatry/fullarticle/208965.

Hughes, John R. "Psychological Effects of Habitual Aerobic Exercise: A Critical Review." *Preventive Medicine* 13, no. 1 (1986): 66–78.

Hutchison, Samantha K., Nigel K. Stepto, Cheryce L. Harrison, Lisa J. Moran, Boyd J. Strauss, and Helena J. Teede. "Effects of Exercise on Insulin Resistance and Body Composition in Overweight and Obese Women with and without Polycystic Ovary Syndrome." *Journal of Clinical Endocrinology and Metabolism* 96, no. 1 (2011): E48–56. https://academic.oup.com/jcem/article-lookup/doi/10.1210/jc.2010-0828.

Kabat-Zinn, Jon. *Wherever You Go, There You Are: Mindfulness Meditation for Everyday Life.* New York: Hyperion, 1994.

Kao, Pai C., Shu-Chu Shiesh, and Ta-Jen Wu. "Serum C-Reactive Protein as a Marker for Wellness Assessment." *Annals of Clinical and Laboratory Science* 36, no. 2 (Spring 2006): 163–69. http://www.annclinlabsci.org/content/36/2/163.full.

Kavey, Neil B. "Stress and Insomnia." *sleepmatters* (Spring 2001). Available online at https://sleepfoundation.org/ask-the-expert/stress-and-insomnia.

Kean, Cornelia. "New Survey Highlights Emotional Toll of Adult Acne." *The Dermatologist* 16, no. 8 (2008). http://www.the-dermatologist.com/article/9048.

Kopera, Daisy, Elisabeth Wehr, and Barbara Obermayer-Pietsch. "Endocrinology of Hirsutism." *International Journal of Trichology* 2, no. 1 (2010): 30–35. http://www.ijtrichology.com/article.asp?issn=0974-7753;year=2010;volume=2;issue=1;spage=30;epage=35;aulast=Kopera.

Levy, Lauren L., and Jason J. Emer. "Female Pattern Alopecia: Current Perspectives." *International Journal of Women's Health* 5 (2013): 541–56. https://www.ncbi.nlm.nih.gov/pmc/articles/PMC3769411/.

Lieber, Charles S. "Alcohol: Its Metabolism and Interaction with Nutrients." *Annual Review of Nutrition* 20 (2000): 395–430.

Lieberman, Harris R., William J. Tharion, Barbara Shukitt-Hale, Karen L. Speckman, and Richard Tulley. "Effects of Caffeine, Sleep Loss, and Stress on Cognitive Performance and Mood during U.S. Navy SEAL Training." *Psychopharmacology* 164, no. 3 (2002): 250–61.

Lipton, Michelle G., Lorraine Sherr, Jonathan Elford, Malcolm H. A. Rustin, and William J. Clayton. "Women Living with Facial Hair: The Psychological and Behavioral Burden." *Journal of Psychosomatic Research* 61, no. 2 (2006): 161–68.

Ludwig, David S., and Jon Kabat-Zinn. "Mindfulness in Medicine." *Journal of the American Medical Association* 300, no. 11 (2008): 1350–52.

Mandal, Ananya. "What Is Ghrelin?" News Medical (website). Last updated September 17, 2014. http://www.news-medical.net/health/What-is-Ghrelin.aspx.

Marcus, Marianne T., and Aleksandra Zgierska. "Mindfulness-Based Therapies for Substance Use Disorders: Part 1 (Editorial)." *Substance Abuse* 30, no. 4 (2009): 263.

Masters, Maria. "12 Facts You Should Know about Ovarian Cysts." *Health.com.* 2015. Accessed May 15, 2017. http://www.health.com/health/gallery/0,,20955242,00.html/view-all.

Matchim, Yaowarat, Jane M. Armer, and Bob R. Stewart. "Effects of Mindfulness-Based Stress Reduction (MBSR) on Health among Breast Cancer Survivors." *Western Journal of Nursing Research* 33, no. 8 (2011): 996–1016.

Mavropoulos, John C., William S. Yancy, Juanita Hepburn, and Eric C. Westman. "The Effects of a Low-Carbohydrate, Ketogenic Diet on the Polycystic Ovary Syndrome: A Pilot Study." *Nutrition and Metabolism* 2 (2005): 35. https://www.ncbi.nlm.nih.gov/pmc/articles/PMC1334192/.

McCluskey, Siobhan E., J. Hubert Lacey, and J. M. Pearce. "Binge-Eating and Polycystic Ovaries." *The Lancet* 340, no. 8821 (1992): 723.

McCook, Judy G., Beth A. Bailey, Stacey L. Williams, Sheeba Anand, and Nancy E. Reame. "Differential Contributions of Polycystic Ovary Syndrome (PCOS) Manifestations to Psychological Symptoms." *Journal of Behavioral Health Services and Research* 42, no. 3 (2015): 383–94.

McCulloch, Fiona. "Does PCOS Make Your Brain More Hungry?" White Lotus Naturopathic Clinic and Integrated Health (website). July 22, 2014. http://www.whitelotusclinic.ca/blog/dr-fiona-nd/hunger-pcos-brain-insulin/.

National Institute of Child Health and Human Development. "Are There Disorders or Conditions Associated with PCOS?" Accessed May 11, 2017. https://www.nichd.nih.gov/health/topics/PCOS/conditioninfo/Pages/conditions-associated.aspx.

National Institute of Mental Health. "Any Anxiety Disorder among Adults." National Institutes of Health. Accessed April 19, 2017. https://www.nimh.nih.gov/health/statistics/prevalence/any-anxiety-disorder-among-adults.shtml.

———. "Dysthymic Disorder among Adults." Accessed May 12, 2017. https://www.nimh.nih.gov/health/statistics/prevalence/dysthymic-disorder-among-adults.shtml.

Nestler, Eric J., Steven E. Hyman, David A. Holtzman, and Robert C. Malenka, eds. "Neural and Neuroendocrine Control of the Internal Milieu." In *Molecular Neuropharmacology: A Foundation for Clinical Neuroscience*, 248–59. New York: McGraw-Hill Medical, 2009.

Otto, Michael, and Jasper A. J. Smits. *Exercise for Mood and Anxiety: Proven Strategies for Overcoming Depression and Enhancing Well-Being*. New York: Oxford University Press, 2011.

Pearson, Aria. "Youthful Infertility Balanced by Late-Blooming Ovaries." *New Scientist*, February 25, 2009. https://www.newscientist.com/article/mg20126973-700-youthful-infertility-balanced-by-late-blooming-ovaries/.

Pearson, Sue, Mike Schmidt, George Patton, Terry Dwyer, Leigh Blizzard, Petr Otahal, and Alison Venn. "Depression and Insulin Resistance: Cross-Sectional Associations in Young Adults." *Diabetes Care* 33, no. 5 (2010): 1128–33. https://doi.org/10.2337/dc09-1940.

Peckham, Carol. "Medscape Physician Compensation Report 2016." Medscape (website), April 1, 2016. http://www.medscape.com/features/slideshow/compensation/2016/public/overview.

Primary Care Dermatology Society. "Hirsutism." Last modified May 29, 2017. http://www.pcds.org.uk/clinical-guidance/hirsutism.

Pruthi, Gavneet K., and Nandita Babu. "Physical and Psychosocial Impact of Acne in Adult Females." *Indian Journal of Dermatology* 57, no. 1 (2012): 26–29. http://www.e-ijd.org/article.asp?issn=0019-5154;year=2012;volume=57;issue=1;spage=26;epage=29;aulast=Pruthi.

Quinn, Molly, Kanade Shinkai, Lauri Pasch, Lili Kuzmich, Marcelle Cedars, and Heather Huddleston. "Prevalence of Androgenic Alopecia in Patients with Polycystic Ovary Syndrome and Characterization of Associated Clinical and Biochemical Features." *Fertility and Sterility* 101, no. 4 (2014): 1129–34. http://www.fertstert.org/article/S0015-0282(14)00033-8/fulltext.

Raja-Khan, Nazia, Katrina Agito, Julie Shah, Christy M. Stetter, Theresa S. Gustafson, Holly Socolow, Allen R. Kunselman, Diane K. Reibel, and Richard S. Legro. "Mindfulness-Based Stress Reduction for Overweight/Obese Women with and without Polycystic Ovary Syndrome: Design and Methods of a Pilot Randomized Controlled Trial." *Contemporary Clinical Trials* 41 (2015): 287–97.

Rasgon, Natalie, and Shana Elman. "When Not to Treat Depression in PCOS with Antidepressants." *Current Psychiatry* 4, no. 2 (February 2005): 47–60. http://www.mdedge.com/currentpsychiatry/article/66214/depression/when-not-treat-depression-pcos-antidepressants.

Rathnayake, Deepani, and Rodney Sinclair. "Innovative Use of Spironolactone as an Antiandrogen in the Treatment of Female Pattern Hair Loss." *Dermatologic Clinics* 28, no. 3 (2010): 611–18.

Rocco, A., P. Falaschi, G. Perrone, P. Pancheri, M. Rosa, and L. Zichella. "Psychoneuroendocrine Aspects of Polycystic Ovary Syndrome." *Journal of Psychosomatic Obstetrics and Gynecology* 12, no. 2 (1991): 169–79.

Rosen, Larry. "Relax, Turn Off Your Phone, and Go to Sleep." *Harvard Business Review*, August 31, 2015. https://hbr.org/2015/08/research-shows-how-anxiety-and-technology-are-affecting-our-sleep.

Ruper, Stephani. "Paleo and PCOS." *Paleo for Women* (blog), May 5, 2012. http://paleoforwomen.com/paleo-and-pcos/.

Sam, Susan. "Obesity and Polycystic Ovary Syndrome." *Obesity Management* 3, no. 2 (2007): 69–73. https://www.ncbi.nlm.nih.gov/pmc/articles/PMC2861983/.

Shapiro, Shauna L., Linda E. Carlson, John A. Astin, and Benedict Freedman. "Mechanisms of Mindfulness." *Journal of Clinical Psychology* 62, no. 3 (2006): 373–86.

Sharifi, Faranak, Sahar Mazloomi, Reza Hajihosseini, and Saideh Mazloomzadeh. "Serum Magnesium Concentrations in Polycystic Ovary Syndrome and Its Association with Insulin Resistance." *Gynecological Endocrinology* 28, no. 1 (2012): 7–11.

Sinha, Rajita. "The Role of Stress in Addiction Relapse." *Current Psychiatry Reports* 9, no. 5 (2007): 388–95.

Society for Endocrinology. "Luteinising Hormone." *You and Your Hormones* (website). Last updated January 7, 2015. http://www.yourhormones.info/hormones/luteinising_hormone.aspx.

Stojanovich, Ljudmila, and Dragomir Marisavljevich. "Stress as a Trigger of Autoimmune Disease." *Autoimmunity Reviews* 7, no. 3 (2008): 209–13.

Tartakovsky, Margarita. "Top Relapse Triggers for Depression and How to Prevent Them." Psych Central (website). Last reviewed July 17, 2016. https://psychcentral.com/lib/top-relapse-triggers-for-depression-how-to-prevent-them/.

Taylor, Shelley. "Coping Strategies." In collaboration with the Psychosocial Working Group. MacArthur Research Network on Socioeconomic Status and Health (website). Last revised July 1998. http://www.macses.ucsf.edu/research/psychosocial/coping.php.

Teasdale, J. D., Z. Segal, and J. M. G. Williams. "How Does Cognitive Therapy Prevent Depressive Relapse and Why Should Control (Mindfulness) Training Help?" *Behaviour Research and Therapy* 33 (1995): 25–39.

Thich Nhat Hanh. "Five Steps to Mindfulness." Mindful (website). August 23, 2010. https://www.mindful.org/five-steps-to-mindfulness/.

Thomson, Rebecca L., Simon Spedding, and Jonathan D. Buckley. "Vitamin D in the Aetiology and Management of Polycystic Ovary Syndrome." *Clinical Endocrinology* 77, no. 3 (2012): 343–50.

Traub, Michael L. "Assessing and Treating Insulin Resistance in Women with Polycystic Ovarian Syndrome." *World Journal of Diabetes* 2, no. 3 (2011): 33–40. https://www.wjgnet.com/1948-9358/full/v2/i3/33.htm.

Unfer, V., G. Carlomagno, G. Dante, and F. Facchinetti. "Effects of Myo-inositol in Women with PCOS: A Systematic Review of Randomized Controlled Trials." *Gynecological Endocrinology* 28, no. 7 (2012): 509–15.

USC Fertility (website). "Learn Fertility Basics: Human Reproduction Hinges on Female Ovulation." Accessed April 1, 2017. http://uscfertility.org/fertility-treatments/fertility-basics/.

Virsaladze, D. K., K. Natmeladze, I. Topuria, A. Natmeladze, and N. Paichadze. "The Effect of Dopamine on Neuroendocrine Disorders in Women with PCOS under Chronic Stress Conditions." *Endocrine Abstracts* 11 (2006): P597.

Vøllestad, Jon, Børge Sivertsen, and Geir Høstmark Nielsen. "Mindfulness-Based Stress Reduction for Patients with Anxiety Disorders: Evaluation in a Randomized Controlled Trial." *Behavior Research and Therapy* 49, no. 4 (2011): 281–88. http://www.sciencedirect.com/science/article/pii/S0005796711000246.

William Glasser Institute–US "Choice Theory." WGlasser.com. Accessed April 2, 2017. http://www.wglasser.com/the-glasser-approach/choice-theory.

Winch, Guy. "Why We All Need to Practice Emotional First Aid." Filmed November 7, 2014. TEDxLinnaeusUniversity video, 17:24. https://www.ted.com/talks/guy_winch_the_case_for_emotional_hygiene.

Zangeneh, Farideh Zafari, Mina Jafarabadi, Mohammad Mehdi Naghizadeh, Nasrine Abedinia, and Fedyeh Haghollahi. "Psychological Distress in Women with Polycystic Ovary Syndrome from Imam Khomeini Hospital, Tehran." *Journal of Reproduction and Infertility* 13, no. 2 (2012): 111–15. https://www.ncbi.nlm.nih.gov/pmc/articles/PMC3719335/.

Zeidan, F., J. A. Grant, C. A. Brown, J. G. McHaffie, and R. C. Coghill. "Mindfulness Meditation–Related Pain Relief: Evidence for Unique Brain Mechanisms in the Regulation of Pain." *Neuroscience Letters* 520, no. 2 (2012): 165–73.

Index

acanthosis nigricans (AN), 141
acne, 4, 7, 12, 26, 63, 64, 70, 115, 126, 135–38
alcohol, 26, 61, 67, 73
amino acids, 24. *See also* tryptophan
androgenic alopecia, 140–41
androgens, 4, 136, 141. *See also* testosterone
Angelou, Maya, 130
anxiety, 46, 56, 57, 63–77, 80, 92, 117, 124, 127, 128, 131–32, 149, 158
appetite, 8, 57, 61
apps: diet/food-tracking, 19, 20, 28, 31, 32, 99; fitness/workout, 39–40, 43, 85; mindfulness meditation, 76, 117, 118, 132; organization, 147

bariatric surgery, 34–35
binge eating, 2, 8, 21–22, 73, 75–76, 129
birth control pills, 7, 10, 27, 66, 68, 137, 139
BMI, 8
Bodhipaksa, 124
body image, 100–101, 102

carbohydrates (carbs), 7, 17, 18–19, 24–25, 73

cardio, 9, 39–40, 43, 49, 69, 158. *See also* exercise
cholesterol, 13, 25
cognitive behavioral therapy (CBT), 66
cortisol, 9, 56, 61, 63, 69–70, 81–82, 104, 107, 109, 114, 115, 128
cravings, 8, 17, 19, 21, 22, 29, 32, 33, 35, 47, 75, 114, 117, 128
C-reactive protein (CRP), 13, 57
cysts, 4, 6, 137, 138, 142

depression, 46, 57, 64, 79–88, 92, 93, 125, 127, 129, 132, 149
diabetes, 6, 18, 32, 56, 115
diet, 11, 17–35, 133

eating disorders. *See* binge eating
Elrod, Hal, 14
estrogen, 6, 8, 142
exercise, 11, 37–53, 69, 71, 83–87, 92, 97, 98–99, 133. *See also* cardio

fats, 25, 57
fertility, 13. *See also* infertility

generalized anxiety disorder (GAD), 3
ghrelin, 57

About the Author

Kelly Morrow-Baez (a.k.a. the FitShrink) is a licensed professional counselor with a PhD in psychology and more than ten years in practice. As a health-motivation expert, she writes for publications like *Thrive Global* and *Everyday Power Blog*, where she explains how mental health, emotional wellness, and physical health are connected and how you can begin your health journey in a way that is empowered and sustainable.

No stranger to PCOS and weight loss, Kelly went through a seventy-five-pound weight loss after the birth of her second child. She believes the best strategy for achieving healthy weight is neither flashy nor extreme—it's purposeful and consistent. Drawing on her personal and professional experience, she developed a strategy to address the physical symptoms of PCOS and lost the weight, putting all but one of her PCOS symptoms into remission. She believes that lasting weight loss and thriving with PCOS is not a one-size-fits-all endeavor. Instead, she believes that approaching lifestyle change with authenticity is infinitely more sustainable. In her view, consistency is better than intensity.

Kelly has been featured in *Dr. Oz: The Good Life* magazine and has added her expertise to articles in *Forbes*, *Teen Vogue*, and *Parents Magazine*, among others. In addition, she has been on numerous podcasts and radio programs to explain the secret to her wellness approach. She is on a mission to change the way people think about getting healthy.

Kelly is a lifelong equestrian, avid runner, failure in the kitchen, and devoted homeschooling mom. When she's not writing, speaking, or coaching, she enjoys spending time with her polo-playing husband, her two kids, and her collection of dogs, cats, and horses on their farm just outside of Columbus, Georgia.

You can learn more about Kelly Morrow-Baez at http://www.fitshrink .com and join her Facebook group, FitShrink PCOS.

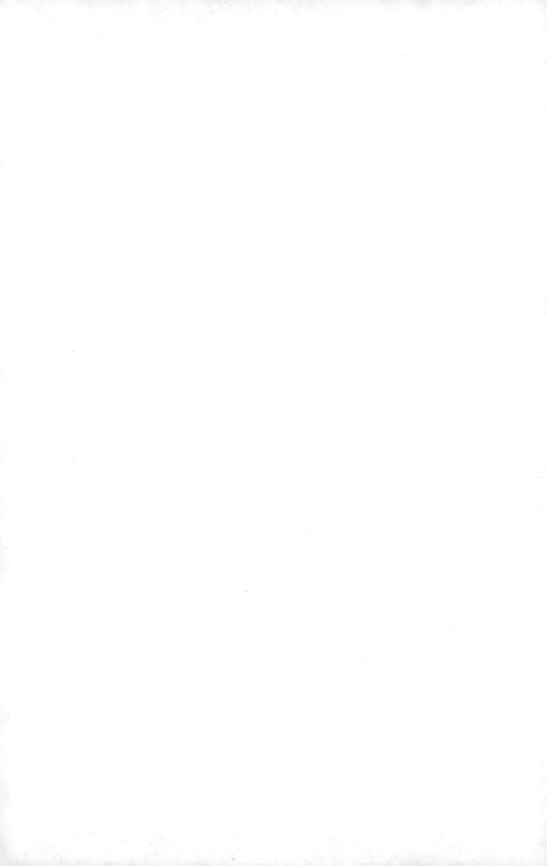